UNIVERSITY OF BIRMINGHAM

Sexual Behaviour
and AIDS in Britain

E G KNOX, C M̵ ̵ ̵ ̵ ̵ ̵, ̵ ̵ SIMON̵ ̵

D1556306

London: HMSO

© Crown copyright 1993
Applications for reproduction
should be made to HMSO
First published 1993

ISBN 0 11 701748 5

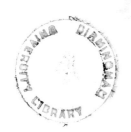

Summary

This report is in three parts. Its objectives are to follow the progress of the AIDS epidemic from its beginning and into the future; and to evaluate alternative preventive options, offering guidance on the best choice and the best manner of implementation. The report employs three classical methods. They include a historical review of the progress of the epidemic to date and of the social and political responses: a field investigation of sexual behaviour and of the potential for sexual transmission in our present day society: and model projections of the future course of the epidemic based on computer simulation. The simulations examine the various interactions between the disease, the sexual behaviour patterns and alternative preventive techniques.

Part 1 – Background and early enquiries

The history of the AIDS epidemic, and of the scientific, social and political responses to it, are of pragmatic as well as general interest. Remarkable scientific advances in understanding the Human Immunovirus (HIV 1) itself, its structure and its biology, and the pathogenesis of the disease to which it gives rise constrast sharply with the confused, contradictory and politically-overburdened approaches to the control of the epidemic process, in many different countries.

Several different methods of extrapolating the course of the current epidemic are described. A distinction drawn between the 'numerical' and 'statistical' techniques employed in the past, and the use of mechanistic transmission models representing natural history processes, sexual behaviour patterns, and virus transmission dynamics within specific populations. Unlike the first group, this last technique offers prospects for testing interventions aimed at its several component processes. Initial computer-simulation exercises showed that transmission via heterosexual contact might in time become the dominant mode. Furthermore the magnitude of the public health problem in this country hinged upon the question whether a viable self-sustaining epidemic will develop among heterosexuals, as it has in some other countries. However, the pragmatic utility of early models was seriously curtailed by a lack of adequate data. It was for this reason that a sexual behaviour survey was designed and executed.

Part 2 – Sexual behaviour in Britain

The survey of sexual behaviour was based upon reports from 1289 male and 1241 female respondents sampled at places of work or similar institutions. The data were gathered through the medium of an anonymous questionnaire, self-completed under 'examination room' conditions, after an introductory explanation from a member of the research team. The main advantages of this form of data collection were the excellent control of responder-bias which it allowed, freedom from the inhibiting presence of family members, and a visible reassurance of absolute anonymity. The questions had overlapping contents, permitting internal checks of consistency: and supplied some potential for the correction of errors.

The questionnaire concentrated especially upon the rates at which first and subsequent partners were acquired at different ages, in different birth cohorts, in the two genders and in different social and demographic groups.

The sample was deliberately biased towards the younger age groups, on which the future course of the epidemic largely depends. Among the men, 83.3 percent had engaged in heterosexual intercourse as had 80.8 percent of the women. Of the men, 6 percent reported homosexual relationships but only 3.4 percent had engaged in anal intercourse. Of the latter group 59 percent had also had female sexual partners. Initiated heterosexual males had had a mean of 6.2 female partners, to date, while initiated females had had 3.9 male partners. This gender difference was probably caused by a combination of technical and selective factors.

The reported sexual careers were incomplete, having been 'intercepted' by the enquiry itself. Further detailed analyses showed that the overall lifetime expectations amounted to about eight sexual partners, both for males and for females. The rate appears to be increasing rapidly, and the most recent sexual cohorts will probably attain a mean total of about twelve sexual partners. There were moderate differences according to different social and demographic characteristics. Frequent partner-changes were associated with less frequent sexual intercourse. There was a strong correlation between age at first intercourse and total subsequent partners, far greater than could be explained by the 'lead time' of an additional year or two of sexual experience. There were also wide individual differences within the various groups.

Among the men, 6.4 percent reported using prostitutes, these encounters representing 4 percent of all heterosexual partnerships reported by men. Heterosexual anal intercourse on at least one occasion was reported by 16.9 percent of the men and 14.2 percent of the women although, for most, this was not a regular practice. Condom usage was found to be greater in the shorter heterosexual relationships and in those with lower monthly intercourse frequencies, but the most striking feature of condom usage was related to the calendar years of the partnerships. Among males engaging in partnerships before 1984, 20 percent used condoms 'usually or always', rising to 47 percent in partnerships starting in 1990/91. The pattern was similar for females. This might be an effect of recent safe-sex media campaigns.

Part 3 – Dynamics of transmission

The dynamics of the transmission of HIV and AIDS were examined using a computer simulation model. It is a 'compartmental' model in which individuals are moved from class to class according to a combination of demographic processes (birth, death, marriage, divorce, remarriage), sexual behaviour data (as assembled and analysed in the above survey) and additional social/sexual behaviour data obtained from the scientific literature; also biological data from other sources on the natural history of HIV infection and levels of infectivity on sexual contact between infected and susceptible persons. The model accommodates different detailed patterns of homosexual and heterosexual behaviour and different levels of partner acquisition, all of which are modified, step by step, according to the current ages of the participants and the years in which they were born. The model can be run for any number of calendar years and it prints out the successive incidences and prevalences of HIV infection, of AIDS itself and of deaths from AIDS at different ages, in the two genders, and in different sexual-behavioural classes.

First experiments with the model demonstrated that the epidemic was extremely sensitive to small variations in estimates of infectivity-on-contact: and much less sensitive to variations in the total numbers of partners. The main effect of the latter variations would be to modify the prevalence of other sexually transmitted diseases and these in turn would increase the infectivity of concurrent HIV. Real-life variations in infectivity through this and other mechanisms successfully explain the difference in epidemic patterns between 'western' and 'third world' communities. In this country, the epidemic pattern appears to be 'co-viable', with autonomous growth among homosexuals, and perhaps the most promiscuous heterosexuals; while continued transmission in the remainder of the population depends upon transfer from the high-risk groups.

Several powerful influences upon growth were uncovered. Varied settings of condom usage exerted powerful effects upon the epidemic projections. By contrast, different settings for the provision and usage of prostitute services exerted relatively minor effects. Indeed, provided that a high proportion of prostitutes could be persuaded to use condoms, the suppression of prostitute services might increase prevalence. Epidemic growth depends upon the extent to which males and females seek partners within their own age groups, or alternatively from a wider age range. Levels of infectivity in the earliest stages of HIV infection are also critical. Effective spread also depends upon the degree to which the most sexually active select their partners from groups with relatively high prevalences of HIV infection. Experiments with hypothetical vaccines showed that programmes directed towards young men were much more successful than those directed towards young women and that a major part of this could be ascribed to the vaccination of the homosexuals. Vaccines which rapidly lose their efficacy are nevertheless extremely useful. Drug treatments which extend the sexually active life of infected people in the later stages of the disease process incurred only a small disbenefit to the rest of the population.

The final chapter outlines the main implications of the findings and formulates an appropriate preventive policy. The main components are based upon the finding that, for the time being, the epidemic in this country remains co-viable (above), and that interventions which influence infectivity – including an increased condom usage – are likely to be far more effective than those which attempt only to influence the current patterns and frequency of heterosexual partner change, or the control of prostitution.

CONTENTS

Part Three – Dynamics of Transmission

PART ONE

Background and Early Enquiries

Chapter 1 – Origins of an Investigation

The scientific and social literature on HIV and AIDS is growing so rapidly that it is now impossible for the individual public health practitioner or public health scientist to read more than a fraction of it. The printed output is already beyond the point at which a single comprehensive digest could be maintained. The scientific endeavour has resolved itself into fields so specialised that those engaged in one may not feel competent to comment upon another. In some of these fields, progress has been truly remarkable. Others leave much to be desired.

Achievements in global monitoring are impressive. The world pandemic is vast and deadly; of that we can be certain. It looks set to be counted as one of the greatest biological disasters ever to befall the human race. Its social, economic and demographic effects will be far reaching. Our knowledge of the virus itself, its structure and its variability, its transcription to a human chromosome, its replication within the cells of the immune system, and the responses of the immune system to its presence are by now well described. The physical facts of the transmission mechanisms from one person to another, and the means of limiting the risk of transmission, are also well understood. There has been some progress in the difficult field of vaccine studies and in the development of drugs for prolonging life and controlling the replication of the virus.

However, our knowledge of the dynamics of epidemic spread within human populations is still rudimentary. The contrast between the limited achievements here, and those in the fields outlined in the previous paragraph, could not be more extreme. The deficiencies apply equally to our knowledge of the epidemic process and to the operational aspects of control. Public health policies in relation to this disease are in many places poorly defined, and sometimes undefined, not to say chaotic. Science and rationality have scarcely been drawn upon in the formulation of control policies and have indeed offered little. Much of the action to date consists of the pursuit of committee procedures, the representation of the rights of individuals and the roles of professional groups, the issue of position statements, and the consumption of paper.

This unsatisfactory state of affairs arises partly from a more general administrative malaise, namely the underdeveloped state of public health practice and the continued inability of politicians and administrators to grapple with the problem of allocating professional responsibilities for public health to those equipped to carry them. It is also a particular problem of this disease, which seems to have engendered a special unwillingness to recognize the facts of the situation, to see the need to designate powers and accountabilities, or to provide sufficient investment and support. Shilts (1), commenting on the epidemic in the USA, noted that 'by 1982 there was already a great deal to ignore'.

There are several subsidiary difficulties, all of which tend to block rational action. The first is the problem of coping emotionally with so terrifying a situation. The second is an unresolved ethical and professional conflict between the priorities to be awarded to the social protection of those already infected, and the physical protection of those not yet infected. The situation has been exacerbated by role-conflicts between public health and clinical practitioners: between medical and non-medical professionals: between scientific advisers to health authorities and the representatives of pressure groups. It has fed political appetites for publicity and for photo-opportunities and for creating profiles of energetic activity dominated by declarations of the need to protect individual rights.

The outcomes of these conflicts have been manifest at many levels – international, national and sub-national – the exact form and balance of the reactions differing in different places. Some countries have adopted isolation measures of some infected persons while others have recoiled from any intrusive measures. In this country, for example, the political reaction to the emergency has included a public denial of the possibility of screening.

These varying reactions can scarcely have been based upon a common appreciation of the deadliness of the hazard, or of the necessities for its control. The formulation of an effective prevention and control policy would seem to be in urgent need of rational analysis and scientific evidence; and an acceptance of the principle that the allocation of resources, priorities and responsibilities should be based upon such evidence. Such acceptance may be less than straightforward in a social environment so overwhelmed by other considerations that it is doubtful whether these primary requirements have yet been recognized.

Context and Objectives of the Present Study

The present report is directed towards these necessities. It describes a short series of investigations contributing to the scientific basis on which an effective control policy might be based. However, we present our findings with some pessimism. There is little evidence within earlier experiences that such evidence might be heeded, or that the mechanisms for controlling the epidemic might be based upon the findings; but the developing severity of the situation may yet force the necessary changes of attitude. (If not, then our report may at least mitigate the risk that future historians, studying the course of the disaster, will visit a judgement of negligence upon public health science.)

The report itself is presented in three parts. The first part provides a resume of the problem as it appeared to us at the time we undertook the research, and of the initial studies which led towards its detailed design. The second and third parts of the report describe the main components of the research itself. The first of these is a descriptive study of selected aspects of sexual behaviour in one part of contemporary Britain; and the second is a description of a computer-based simulation model of the HIV epidemic. This model was designed to predict the form of the epidemic under a range of different plausible assumptions, and to describe its responses to the different decisions and actions which public health practitioners and authorities might take.

Although the three parts of the report are presented seriatim, and although the technical aspects of each are distinct, they were designed as an integrated whole. Each stage of the analysis was necessary for the proper development and interpretation of the others. The first step was the development and application of an equilibrium model, first published in 1986 (2). At this stage the UK epidemic had been recognized for less than three years. The purpose of the model was to predict the general magnitude of the epidemic at its eventual 'steady state' – the stage when deaths from the disease rise to equal the numbers of new cases then being generated. This study reached the alarming conclusion that by the middle of the 21st century there may be 20,000 to 40,000 deaths per annum from AIDS in the UK. The main note of comfort was that the epidemic would be slow to develop. There was still time to collect the necessary data, to refine the predictions, and to devise those policies which would most effectively counter the hazard.

This equilibrium model, like all communicable disease models, was based upon a mix of knowledge and of assumptions concerning contact patterns within affected communities, and estimates of the biological risk of transmission when such contacts occurred. The model and its outcomes were crude and unreliable, demanding refinement and more accurate data; and especially data. On some points relating to sexual behaviour we had almost no data at all, and on others we had to extrapolate gleanings from the Kinsey Report on sexual behaviour (3), whose results were separated from current requirements in the UK by the distance of an ocean, a gap of fifty years, and a social/sexual revolution.

This model exercise revealed not only the paucity of available data and their inappropriateness to the questions now being asked; but it specified which particular items of information were necessary if this approach was to be pursued further. We were able to say, now, what forms of data would be required to justify the effort of developing the model further, and thus provide a rational basis for controlling the epidemic. Indeed, it was this early exercise which determined the design of the sexual behaviour survey which we describe in Part 2 of this report.

The development of an improved predictive model was pursued in parallel, and its general structure was set against the information which we now hoped to collect. In the event, the details and the scale of the available information were limited by practical constraints. This forced further modifications upon the design of the model including both elaborations and simplifications. This, in turn led us to readjust our demands for data.

The original modelling work which led to the present study was conducted without specific funding and it arose as a technical continuation of research already conducted and reported on the epidemiology of cancer of the cervix and its relationship with the transmission of Human Papilloma Virus (HPV) (4, 5). This research had been conducted within a programme of Health Services Research supported by the Department of Health (DoH) and negotiations for support for the new proposals were pursued through the same quarter. Application of this modelling approach to the problem of AIDS was positively encouraged by the Office of the Chief Scientist to the DoH to the extent that we were advised to give it priority at the expense of our other funded research activities. At this point, however, DoH funds relating to AIDS research were redirected from the Chief Scientist's office to a special DoH Research Unit to which epidemiological teams such as our own had no established routes of access; and, shortly afterwards, the financial resources were transferred yet again as the work was contracted out to the Medical Research Council. It was then necessary to restart funding negotiations, and although the necessary financial resources were obtained from the Medical Research Council, we had by then lost two doubling times, as measured on the HIV scale. This delay, together with the uncertainty as to whether we might proceed at all, and our difficulties in estimating what level of funding might be available, supplied the third major constraint upon our approach to the problem, and on the design of the research programme.

The development of a practical working model, the design of the data collecting processes, and the process of seeking financial support were mutually interactive and mutually dependent. They evolved together as part of a complex and changing process with each part responding to the pressures of the others. This is not unusual in applied research and is to some extent unavoidable, but the complexities and circularities were in this case exceptional, consuming a great deal of effort and time. Only the purpose of the research was constant from the beginning.

Chapter 2 – Early Experience of HIV in Great Britain

AIDS was first recognized in the USA in 1981 as a new disease of male homosexuals. The numbers of cases expanded in an explosive manner and by October 1983 more than 2500 cases had been diagnosed by the US Public Health Service (6). The phenomenon which we now know as the 'UK AIDS epidemic' first surfaced in 1982, with 2 cases. In 1983 and 1984 there were 99 recorded cases, with 442 in the next two years, and 1291 in the two years after that (7).

By 1982 the features of the disease had been attributed to a deficiency of the immune system, its transmissibility had been recognized and its viral origin was suspected. This was confirmed through the isolation and characterisation of the virus in 1983 (8, 9) and a serological test for antibodies was available shortly afterwards. Since that time, HIV-disease has been defined primarily on the criterion of the presence of antibodies to the antigenic components of the virus. A comprehensive understanding of the disease-process, expressed in review articles (10, 11), was available by 1985; a truly remarkable rate of scientific progress.

In addition to the explosive nature of the epidemic, there were several features of the illness itself which excited – or variously deadened – social and political responses to it. First, AIDS was incurable; no-one ever recovered from it. Second, the incubation period was prolonged and symptomless, allowing adequate opportunity for onward transmission. Third, although it was at first supposed that only a small proportion of those infected with the virus would develop AIDS, it soon became apparent that this was a false impression arising from the long incubation period; and that the majority of those infected – possibly all – would eventually develop and die from the disease. Fourth, it was a disease associated in the public and political eye with activities regarded by many as depravities, including drug addiction, homosexual anal intercourse, extreme promiscuity and prostitution. In the early days it was seen as a 'disease of social pariahs' (1).

This last factor was a serious inhibition to rational thought and analysis. Discussion required a consideration of practices which many found so repugnant that they were unwilling to enquire into the exact details – of what homosexuals actually *did*, for example – or even to learn or use the necessary vocabularies. In addition as the media began to report the problem, the associations of the disease with third world poverty, and with ghetto conditions in certain western societies, also became clear. Attitudes to the epidemic became linked with differing social policies and political ideologies; and with contrasting attitudes towards disciplinary and assistance-orientated public-health measures. These conflicts were nowhere more obvious than in relation to drug related transmission, and prostitution, themselves often linked.

The homosexual groups themselves took constructive action to limit the spread of the disease among them. However, they also defended their behaviour patterns and their social rights to pursue them with sufficient vigour to aggravate some of the public and political approbations. As a result, a major part of the subsequent discussion became focused upon threats of discrimination and actual discrimination and upon the protection of potential victims arising from social attitudes at work, disadvantages in seeking insurance or mortgages, and in other situations. These discussions were not without benefit. They raised real moral, ethical and legal issues and forced a depth of thinking not often undertaken in relation to other public health topics (12, 13, 14, 15, 16, 17, 18, 19, 20, 21, 22); but in some quarters these discussions raised the temperature rather than the clarity of the argument.

The consequences of these confrontations included the a priori political exclusion of screening as a public health option in the UK: a denial of the possibility of notification and the barring of proposed public health surveillance measures using available blood specimens. This was later modified to a grudging admission of the necessity but with scientifically crippling provisos relating to identification. Finally, both in this country and in the USA, funding was withdrawn from large-scale sexual behaviour surveys which had been undertaken or were planned in order to measure the social patterns which had determined the course of the epidemic, and in order to project its future course. It appeared that the questions which had to be asked were just too much for the political stomach.

Much of this chaotic thinking was undocumented, pursuing circular tracks within the confines of committees, and seeking compromises among the minefields of professional and political role conflicts. This occurred in district and regional strategy committees as well as at government level, much of it hidden from public view, but appearing occasionally in explicit form within the framework of official guidelines, and in generally dogmatic quasi-ethical formulations of various corporate bodies.

The situation generated and partly resulted from a measure of wishful thinking – the notion that it might not happen here, that it might go away, that it does not actually exist, that HIV is not the cause of AIDS; and that an effective treatment or vaccine will shortly be discovered. Many found a deadly epidemic of such magnitude and stealth to be literally unthinkable.

Finally, and perhaps most fundamentally in the UK, AIDS had encountered a public health service in a serious state of disrepair. Public Health practitioners had suffered several transmutations of their job descriptions and responsibilities – notably in 1974 and 1982. Responsibility for the public health was scattered across Health Districts, Health Regions, Local Government Authorities, government departments and the Public Health Laboratory Service (PHLS). The PHLS had a well organized national structure – sufficient to have successfully resisted and recovered from a government proposal for its dissolution – but there was no longer a well-structured public health organization to draw upon its services. Public Health practitioners were employed in many separate organizations within the NHS and elsewhere, but there was no unifying structure. These difficulties had been recognized, and the definition of the public health role was at that time under review by the Acheson Committee (23) but no corrective formulations were yet available: or likely to be acted upon for some time.

The control of communicable diseases had fallen by default to a subsidiary position. Indeed, responsibility for the control of communicable diseases still rested, legally, with the Local Government Authorities who had earlier supplied one of the three arms of the 'tripartite' system which had been dissolved in 1974. This responsibility had become identified, largely, with the control of food poisoning. For the remainder, there was no natural locus of leadership. Unscheduled outbreaks of disease – for example legionnaires disease – resulted typically in confusion concerning professional responsibilities, and delays in recognizing that there was an epidemic at all. Global responsibilities for communicable disease control had become inverted to the extent that the only central office engaged in such duties, The Communicable Disease Surveillance Centre (CDSC) had developed as a subset of the laboratory service. On top of this, the responsibilities of Public Health practitioners and the nature of Public Health science were widely misunderstood, even among professionals.

It is also a fact that the theoretical basis of Public Health science and of Public Health practice is weak. The strong theoretical basis of clinical medicine, supplied by a century or more of intensive research in physiology and pathology, is simply not available in this field. Furthermore, formal mathematical modelling, the necessary basis of modern Public Health planning, is well calculated to close the minds of all but a few. Many regard it as a private recreation, tangential to real issues. It would be difficult to find any general recognition of the fact that modelling is the necessary basis of prediction: that prediction is the necessary basis of planning and control: and that modelling is therefore the necessary basis of any rational approach to controlling this epidemic.

Those who write the history of this disease will be intrigued by the contrasts which it displays: the implacable deadliness of the biological hazard: the still-primitive but rapidly-developing scientific foundation for understanding, predicting and controlling epidemics: the urgent need to allocate resources, powers and responsibilities for its control: and a disregard of all of them within a social response dominated by other concerns.

Chapter 3 – Extrapolation and Prediction

The first approach to predicting the form and the growth rate of the epidemic was through extrapolation. At its simplest, numbers of new cases are plotted on graph paper year by year and the curve is projected forward. The early stages of many epidemics are logarithmic, like the curve of bacterial growth in a culture-broth. This is to say that the numbers increase by a fixed *ratio* each year, rather than by a fixed amount.

There are good theoretical reasons why this should be so. Each case gives rise to an average of 'R' other cases during the time taken for the original case to die or recover. The value 'R' is called the Reproductive Ratio. If 'R' is greater than 1.0, then each original case is replaced, with interest. If 'R' is less than 1.0, then the replacement is incomplete and the epidemic declines and eventually dies out. If there is in fact a rising epidemic, as there is for HIV, then we know that 'R' must be greater than 1.0.

A curve based upon a constant rate of increase tends eventually to infinity, as in Malthusian population growth; which is to say that in the long term it cannot be maintained and that at some stage the rate of growth must level off. In the short-term, however, this pattern of growth is a reasonable assumption, especially where the epidemic seems indeed to be following such a curve. It is on this basis that a limited extrapolation has been justified. The graphical extrapolation can then be drawn on semi-logarithmic graph paper, where it is represented as a straight line.

In fact, the mechanism of the AIDS epidemic is far more complex than the bacterial growth analogy, and contains several separate epidemic components. They include an epidemic among male homosexuals, an epidemic among drug users, a heterosexual epidemic, an epidemic among haemophiliacs and an epidemic in new born babies. In addition to local exponential growth in each separate curve, each progressing at a different rate, there is the complication of geographical spread, with progressive seeding of areas remote from the original centre; and the independent take-off of new epidemics, in each risk group, in each of these new sites. The aggregate of these separate curves is not necessarily logarithmic at all. Biological diversity adds another problem and early estimations of growth rates were biased because of over-representation (among known cases of AIDS) of those with the most rapidly progressive disease, and those with high-risk behaviour. A further distortion arose, in the opposite direction, through delayed reporting; as each year has passed, optimists have grasped hopefully at an apparent 'most recent' tailing-off in the growth rate. As each next year arrived, the late registrations dashed these hopes, only for them to be revived at the next annual count. To add a perverse complication, there is evidence since 1990 of a genuine reduction in the rate of increase, together with indicators of changes in the sexual behaviour of high risk groups, as reflected in a dip in the presentation of new cases of gonorrhoea. There is a counter suggestion that both of these represent not so much a reduction of sexual transmissions as a fear of HIV testing, and a reluctance to seek treatment. Yet another possibility has been suggested, namely that AIDS-onsets are being postponed through treatment of known HIV-positives with zidovudine.

The uncertainties of logarithmic projection are therefore clear, but there is a corroborative form of extrapolation consisting of the transfer of growth rates observed in one country, to another. Both in numbers and proportions the USA is further down the epidemic path than any other 'Western' country. Within Europe, both France and Switzerland are ahead of Great Britain. It has generally been assumed, with appropriate reservations, that if one country can locate its position on another country's growth curve, then it is likely to follow the same path over the next time-interval. The reservations arise because some countries exhibit a predominance of intravenous drug user transmissions (Spain, Italy, Scotland), while others exhibit an excess of male homosexual transmission (Netherlands, USA), while in others – mainly countries in Central Africa – the primary mode of transmission is heterosexual. The method of international analogy can also be used more locally, and once a local City or Region has become infected then it can be supposed that it will follow the patterns already observed in other Cities and Regions. This also demands circumspection. Glasgow and Liverpool have not followed Edinburgh in its needle-born epidemic, despite similar levels of IV drug-usage.

International data are not always reliable. It is widely believed that some countries suppressed dissemination of the true statistics of the disease for political and economic (tourist industry) reasons, while in others the statistical services are less than competent or disabled by political pressures or lack of resources. More emphasis has been placed, possibly, upon the non-comparability of different countries rather than their similarities. For example, the predominantly heterosexual spread in Central and Eastern Africa has been attributed to a prolific use of prostitutes and the widespread prevalence of other ulcerative genital diseases. It is a proven fact that the presence of ulcers and of pus cells increases the risk of heterosexual transmission of HIV, and this has been widely quoted in support of hopeful and perhaps wishful assumptions that heterosexual transmission will not be a major problem in Britain. Another international difference, within Europe, arises from the varying proportions of 'imported' cases, a particular problem in countries with recent African colonies (e.g. Belgium) or widespread use of foreign travel (e.g. Sweden).

There is a third way of extrapolating from the present to the future. The growth pattern in AIDS deaths follows the growth of numbers of clinical presentations, after a lag-interval of one or perhaps two years. Numbers of known cases should in principle permit a more extended projection of the deaths, than do the current deaths themselves. However, most countries do not know how many AIDS cases there are and the deaths continue to provide the more reliable statistic. In the United Kingdom, for example, the possibility of notification was pre-empted politically. Although returns of known new cases reported by clinicians are collected centrally, local lists are assembled under imposed difficulties without the possibility of excluding duplicates, or relating clinical reports to laboratory tests, or specifying risk groups, or identifying relationships between different cases, or exact geographical locations. Furthermore, the emotional and clinical difficulties of handling the situation have led to diagnostic fudging. HIV positives with symptoms arising from their disease have often been labelled as 'AIDS-Related Complex' (ARC), and the diagnosis delayed or avoided. Even the deaths from AIDS are sometimes classified to other causes. For example, there has been a recent increase in deaths from 'pneumonia' in young men.

Just as the curve of AIDS deaths follows the numbers of AIDS cases after an interval of a year or two, so the numbers of AIDS cases follow the numbers of HIV infections after an interval of perhaps 8 to 12 years. The AIDS cases and AIDS deaths occurring now are the consequences of infections acquired 8 to 12 years ago. Unfortunately, these numbers are hidden from us and certain political decisions are well calculated to see that they remain so. A recent Secretary of State for Health barred the possibility of screening, in consistent accord with the negative policy on notification. A more recent appointee has been encouraging people to 'come forward for testing' but it is not clear whether this implies a change of policy or is a simple reflection of muddle. For the present, the relationship between infections and clinical cases have to be calculated in reverse. Current numbers of infective persons are estimated by 'back projection' from known numbers of clinical cases and deaths. This depends upon a knowledge of the natural history of the disease, which is uncertain, but once the back projection has been carried out it is possible then to project the epidemic forward, through the present time and on towards the future (24, 25, 26, 27, 28, 29, 30, 31, 32, 33, 34, 35, 36, 37, 38). It is an uncertain art.

There are major statistical difficulties with this approach. The outcomes depend critically upon small variations in estimates of the duration of the natural history, its variability, and the rates at which incidence and prevalence are in fact increasing. For example, if AIDS has a mean interval of ten years from infection to presentation, and if the growth of new infections has continued to follow the growth of clinical AIDS – doubling each year – then the ratio between new infections and clinical cases in recent years will be about 2^{10} – that is about 1000:1. A population with a thousand cases in one year, will have generated a million new HIV infections in the same year. The facts for the UK, such as they are, suggest that this cannot possibly be true.

In the UK, between October 1989 and September 1990, there were recorded 1063 new cases of AIDS acquired through homosexual or heterosexual intercourse or injecting drug use (39). Only 15,000 infecteds had so far been identified (in September 1990). Detected cases are only the tip of an iceberg, but evidence available from serological surveys (40, 41) shows that the total number of infected persons must be much lower than the exponential calculations suggest. Known non-clinical HIV-positives are essentially limited to those who have received infected blood products, those in high risk groups, those in previous contact with other infected persons, and those attending STD clinics. The explanation of the discrepancy probably lies in the powerful geographical concentrations of cases and their confinement to particular districts and particular high risk groups such as IV drug users and male homosexuals. These localised groups are approaching HIV saturation. Exponential growth of new infections has tailed off through depletion of the remaining susceptibles, without having so far generated a similar epidemic growth in other groups and in other districts. The lesson to be drawn is that this form of extrapolation, like the other forms, is dangerously inadequate.

Chapter 4 – Next Questions

Unless a safe and economic cure for HIV infection can be developed, then the primary health objective must be to limit new infections with HIV. Likewise, the primary research requirement must be to clarify those social and biological questions whose answers will help us limit the rate at which uninfected people become infected.

We must at the same time provide facilities for counselling and treating established cases, and we must plan and supply resources to do so in sufficient time to meet the growing demand. However, where there is competition for resources a higher priority must be given to the primary preventive objective: an infection prevented now saves many infections in the course of the following years and reduces the size of the ultimate disaster. It is of course a silent disaster. The effects are not manifest as a visible epidemic until several years later. By the time it reached levels sufficient to cause real concern, if no action had been taken, it would be too advanced to be averted.

Koch (42) has drawn an analogy with other communicable disease agents, part of whose evolutionary and survival 'strategy' is to alter behaviour in their hosts. The common cold makes its victims sneeze, the threadworm makes its host itch (and scratch), and the rabies virus makes its victims bite. Koch has suggested that the success of viruses with long latent intervals must be attributed partly to their epidemiological silence, and the manner in which they deaden and delay the prospects for an effective public response.

How is an effective control process to be accomplished? It is not possible at present to answer this question. The necessary actions at the individual level are clear enough – limitation of partner-changes, avoidance of high-risk sexual practices, use of condoms, and avoidance of needle sharing. However, if public health programmes are to go beyond the screening of donated blood and general exhortation directed towards the public at large, then we shall have to learn how to target our limited resources effectively. We shall then have to measure their effectiveness and to modify policies, programmes and investments in the light of the measured performance. This is a daunting task. Few of the necessities are in place and we shall have to ask many questions, many of them year after year. For example . . .

> 1) How many cases of HIV-infecteds are there now; what is its prevalence?
>
> 2) At what rate are new cases occurring; what is the incidence?
>
> 3) How are the infected persons distributed geographically, by sexual behaviour type, by age group, by sex, by ethnic group and by social and educational group?
>
> 4) Who is infecting whom? What for example is the relative importance of needle transmission, homosexual transmission, heterosexual transmission and maternal/fetal transmission and how quickly is the picture changing?

5) What are the frequencies, within the population, of different forms of sexual partnership, including homosexual partnerships, heterosexual partnerships, multiple simultaneous partnerships, and relationships between homosexual/bisexual men and heterosexual women? How long do these partnerships last and how quickly do they change? Do they overlap, or are they separated by gaps? At what rates are new partners taken up and old partners given up?

6) How do the partner-switching patterns, and the contact rates within partnerships vary according to age, birth cohort, duration of partnership, social class, ethnic group and drug usage?

7) What are the frequencies of intercourse within homosexual and heterosexual partnerships? Within multiple partnerships, and between homosexual men and heterosexual women? What are the mean values and what is the distribution about these means?

8) How infectious is the disease in its different stages in these various contact groups? What are the magnitudes of the risks associated with each type of contact?

9) What is the natural history of HIV infection? What are the mean durations and distributions of sojourn within the various stages? To what extent does infectivity change in the different stages of the disease?

10) To what extent would different behaviour-modifications, effected through targeted health education, and with different projected efficacies in different groups, inhibit the growth of the epidemic? What will be the relative effectiveness and the combined effectiveness of altered sexual behaviour (i.e. contact rates and rates of partner change) and an increased use of condoms?

11) How responsive are the different social and sexual behaviour groups to general health education approaches, and to targeted health education?

12) What would be the effects of population-wide screening followed by highly-targeted advice on sexual behaviour; of selective screening in high-risk groups such as male homosexuals and drug users; of contact tracing of HIV positives, with similar educational interventions; of contact tracing of those with gonorrhoea or other STD's; and of selective screening and selective quarantine?

13) What is the part played by male and by female prostitution in the spread of the disease, especially prostitution linked with drug usage, and what measure of control might be obtained through regulating prostitution or through enforced registration and supervision and screening of prostitutes, or through attempted suppression, or through selective pensioning or quarantine?

14) What is the likely effectiveness of providing free replacement of needles and syringes for drug addicts, either in the context of drug clinics or through liberal 'no questions asked' dispensing schemes? What are the effects of police action? What

would be the effects of supplying drugs to addicts in return for medical supervision and screening?

15) What would be the effect of a vaccine delivered to the whole of the sexually active population, or alternatively to specific risk groups, or specific ages, or to only one of the sexes, or to those attending for the treatment of sexually transmitted diseases, or to prostitutes? What would be the effect in each of these circumstances of a vaccine which was only partially effective, or which was effective only for a limited time?

16) What would be the effect of treatments – drugs or antibodies or T-cell transfusions, for example – which prolong the lives of HIV positive people, improve their health, and extend the scale of their sexual contacts? What would be the effect if such treatment reduced the infectivity of HIV disease by some measurable amount?

17) What investments are necessary and what returns can be expected from them? Can the control-process be handled from within the existing pattern of health care organisation and within existing legal powers? If not, then what kind of organisation must be established and what additional powers must be sought ?

Questions of Different Kinds

The above questions are mainly epidemiological in character but they are of two distinct types. First, there are questions which can in principle be answered through direct observation and enquiry – for example, information on current prevalences and incidences, or patterns of change of sexual partner at different ages, in different cohorts and in different social groups. The other class of question can be answered only through projections from the past and present towards the future. We ask both for unconditional and conditional predictions. What is going to happen? What will happen IF . . . ? For example, what would happen if behaviour patterns changed, if treatment prolonged sexually active life, if a vaccine became available, if health education could achieve a reduction of 10 percent in heterosexual partner changes . . . and so on.

Questions about the future require a quite different approach; they can not be answered by field-enquiries. This is a fundamental point. Conditional and unconditional predictions demand the development, the validation and the application of adequate models. This is a fundamental requirement of all scientific approaches and the rules are no different for public health science and public health practice than they are for aircraft design, weather forecasting or astrophysics. Furthermore, extrapolation models such as those described earlier will not suffice for this purpose. They do not supply the possibilities of simulated interventions, necessary for testing alternative control measures. For this purpose we need quantitative sexual transmission models, and the models must be 'parametrised' using the observations derived from the first class of questions – those depending upon direct observation. At a later stage we might also hope to test and validate these models against observations relating to other sexually transmitted diseases, modifying the disease-related parameters, but leaving the behavioural characteristics in place.

The parametrisation of these models, and perhaps even the structure of the models, must be related to those specific populations where intervention is proposed, and the control systems which are to implement it. The biological characteristics of the disease are likely to remain more or less constant between different populations – provided that we take into account such factors as ulcerative STD's – so we can use biological data from other populations with substantial experience of these matters. However, we cannot transfer social data from other populations into our own predictive mechanisms without first ascertaining the extent and manner in which our own social and behavioural data differ from theirs. Nor can we transfer social behavioural data for our own society, where monogamous marriage is the norm, to another where polygamous marriage is the norm. Effective local action is uniquely dependent upon local social-sexual data, upon models reflecting local patterns of sexual behaviour, and upon models incorporating locally-feasible interventions.

Chapter 5 – Equilibrium Models and Dynamic Models

Model making is not an optional activity. Models are the *only* way of making predictions, conditional or unconditional. We may use good models or bad models, intuitive models or mathematical models, diagrammatic (iconic) models or computer models. There is a choice there. But we *must* use models. Models are not, as is sometimes believed, a therapeutic activity for those with no data and nothing much to do. They are the necessary tool for extrapolating from any pattern of observations to any other situation and for predicting the future on the basis of observations already made. Facts are a necessary precursor – but not a substitute. In the future, with which we are necessarily concerned, there are indeed no facts at all. Facts are confined to the past.

Model-making for communicable diseases has a long but sparse history; a history not noted for its pragmatic utility in disease control. The first recorded mathematical model – relating to the spread of measles in a residential school – was devised by En'ko, in 1889 (43). The work was entered for an MD thesis in the University of St. Petersburg. En'co no doubt dumbfounded his examiners, who probably did not understand it, but he gained his MD! The same problem was tackled by Hamer in London in 1906 and Ross developed the mass action principle in relation to malaria in 1908 (44, 45, 46, 47, 48).

The subsequent history of communicable disease modelling, like these initial essays, has often appeared as an exercise in mathematical relationships rather than an attempted solution of a real public health problem. Until recently, those engaged in developing the theory found a more receptive readership among mathematicians and other theoreticians than among those in public health practice (49,50). The essential technical stimulus to practical population modelling was the advent of the computer. The earliest explorations and applications were pioneered by Elveback in the USA (51).

Since then, mathematical modelling has found a more extended place within public health control systems, and has sometimes provided essential policy guidance – for example in the control of schistosomiasis and onchocerciasis; but the applications are still sporadic. Different workers have addressed problems relating to the spread of tuberculosis (52), infective diarrhoea (53), typhoid (54) and other bacterial diseases (55), influenza, rabies, poliomyelitis and other virus diseases (56, 57, 58), hookworm (59), and even rumours (60). Substantial advances have recently been made in the formal mathematical representation of infectious transmission, and their extension to evaluate preventive interventions (61, 62, 63). These and similar models have been used successfully to predict the effects of alternative vaccination programmes for influenza, measles and rubella (64, 65, 66, 67, 68), whooping cough (69) and tetanus (70). They have also proved invaluable in agricultural pest control. Modelling has also found a useful place in predicting the effects of alternative public health policies concerned with non-communicable diseases; for example, deployments of screening services for the control of cervical cancer and breast cancer (71, 72, 73).

Until recently, and with one or two exceptions, their application to the control of sexually transmitted diseases has been less than fruitful. Early models by Constable (74) and by Reynolds and Chan (75) established the compartmental structure of such models and showed how they could be 'solved' mathematically through representing the transfers between one disease state and another in the form of differential equations. The second of these studies was focussed upon control and directed towards pragmatic application. Yorke, Hethcote and Nold (76) and Lajmanovich and Yorke (77) developed this process, devising models for gonorrhoea which they used in order to determine optimal policies for contact tracing within a specific service. They tried to show whether it was better to invest in tracing the contacts of infected men or of infected women, and whether to concentrate upon contacts prior to the infection, or afterwards. The result was perhaps obvious in qualitative terms – namely to give priority to tracing the prior contacts of infected men. However, they were also able to quantify their results and provide valuable economic comparisons of the projected costs and benefits of the alternative approaches.

The epidemiology of cancer of the cervix, and of its pre-cancerous pathology, has also been represented as a sexual transmission model (4,5). The epidemiology of human papilloma virus (HPV) in its various strains is an essential plank of such models. These models have improved our understanding of the recent growth and the changing age-specific prevalence of pre-invasive lesions, presumptively due to HPV, and their dependence upon the greater rates of change of sexual partners in more recent birth cohorts of men and of women. In this case, as with HIV, we are dealing with a chronic and chronically infective condition, as opposed to the acute and transitorily infective processes involved with gonorrhoea.

The essential characteristics of the behaviour of a communicable disease, and of the structure of a model designed to represent it, depend less upon whether it is acute or chronic, as upon its capacity to generate immunity. For the acute immunising diseases, the accelerating epidemic leads to a progressive depletion of the susceptibles, reducing the reproductive ratio (R) below unity, thus causing the epidemic to decline. However, before the disease finally disappears, the pool of susceptibles is replenished with the birth of new children; or, in some cases, by the waning of a transient immunity or an antigenic change in the organism. Another epidemic then follows.

Sexually transmitted diseases seldom elicit immunity. Their survival strategies depend upon their abilities to evade the host's immune system. Most of them cause chronic diseases, infectious over many years – at least in some of the affected persons. In such infections the depletion and replenishment of susceptibles plays a relatively minor role. In a homogeneous population where 'R' is greater than unity, the disease can spread until almost everyone is infected, subject only to a small proportional loss and replenishment through death and recruitment. Alternatively, if the reproductive ratio is less than 1.0 – say in a sexually abstemious sub-population – then the disease will disappear altogether.

In practice, a 'mid-position' quasi-equilibrium is frequently attained because populations are not homogeneous. It is this, rather than the periodic depletion and replenishment of susceptibles, which determines and characterises the epidemic pattern of a chronic sexually transmitted disease. That is, there are some groups, some zones, some age groups . . . for example . . . where the spread of the disease proceeds towards saturation; and there are other groups which, if isolated from the saturated groups, would see the disease proceed to extinction. The survival of the disease, exhibiting a finite and more-or-less steady prevalence – which is what we observe in sexually transmitted diseases – depends upon the existence of the two kinds of groups, side by side, with a steady trickle of infection from the saturated to the unsaturated, and the maintenance of an overall equilibrium for the population as a whole. Behavioural heterogeneity is of the essence, in understanding these diseases. It is also the essential characteristic of any realistic model.

Several simple models of HIV, developed in recent years, have mimicked transmission patterns and epidemic growth within confined circumstances, for example within male homosexual relationships (78), or in heterosexual partnerships (79). However, the above considerations suggest that our best hope for developing a realistic model for the whole population is to devise a set of partly independent models for each sexual behaviour type, but where each type interacts with the other types. These interactions are represented as an inter-group contact-matrix. Within each behaviour-type there is a further level of heterogeneity for different levels of sexual activity; and yet other levels for different ages, different ethnic groups, different social classes and different birth cohorts. This places great demands upon the complexity of the design process, upon the detail of the data necessary for setting the parameters of the model, and upon the need to validate outcomes against observations.

Different investigators have tried to cope with these constraints in different ways. Some have developed the theoretical and mathematical aspects of an infectious growth model in considerable detail, uncovering additional complexities and additional predictive difficulties (80, 81, 82). Other analysts (83, 84) have tended to ameliorate this explosive growth of complexity, arguing that beyond a certain point these refinements possibly add little to the predictive value of less elaborate systems. These are of course dangerous arguments; it is never possible to say, until sensitivities to particular details have been tested, that any new facet of the argument may not be critical. In the meantime, lacking adequate data, or indeed an adequate computer implementation, most of these authors have avoided making numerical predictions. A particularly useful review by Doust (85) of predictive exercises – part of an annotated bibliography covering many different aspects of HIV infection – listed 84 publications on this theme between 1986 and 1990. Following our own 1986 paper (2) only 2 of the 84 were based explicitly upon mechanistic compartmental models involving multiple behaviour types, and from which numerical estimates were attempted. One additional paper, not included in the above review (86), tackled the problem of linked risk groups and illustrated the importance of inter-group transmission by imposing an experimental mutual isolation of homosexuals and heterosexuals. However, the study remains essentially theoretical without concrete numerical predictions, whether conditional or unconditional.

Most of the difficulties arose from lack of adequate data; and the difficulties of assembling the necessary information are indeed formidable. However, we ourselves took the view that this was the only technical route which seemed ultimately capable of providing a practical predictive tool and a basis for testing the likely efficacy of preventive interventions *before* they were put in place. It was this consideration, combined with a lack of adequate information, which had led us to adopt the strategy of simplifying our initial model (2) to predict only the equilibrium position which might be reached after a period of many years. It did not attempt to predict the rate at which the equilibrium would be approached or say more than approximately when the steady state would be reached. The less specific predictions attempted by this model required less specific data inputs. The predictions were also explicitly dependent upon particular rates of change of sexual partnerships in different sexual behaviour classes which had been derived only roughly from a range of inadequate sources; in particular the Kinsey report. Depending upon the assumption that these behaviour patterns would not change, it was estimated that in the United Kingdom there might eventually be 20,000 to 40,000 deaths per annum. The expected growth rate was slow: and slowest of all among the heterosexual population. The equilibrium position might be reached by about 2030 AD. The model also predicted that a vaccine, even if it were partly effective and partly taken up, would be extremely effective. Not only are the immunised persons themselves protected, but they occupy the now-ineffective attentions of infected persons. There is an analogy here with pest control through the sterilisation and release of parasitic flies. The model also predicted that educational activities designed to reduce frequencies of partner-switching would be less than effective if used alone, but might be more effective where they were used as an adjunct to a vaccine programme.

In pragmatic public health terms, the model itself was less than successful. So far as is known, it played no part in any policy formulations and was never referenced in any official publications. Its predictions were perhaps too expensive to contemplate and it held out little hope that the current health education policy would have much effect. Its predictions were also unreliable – although no less so than others – in that the data on which the predictions depended were themselves unreliable. Probably the main value of that model, at that stage, lay in the 'sensitivity analyses' which it permitted. These analyses explored the extent to which the predictions depended upon variations and uncertainties of the different parameters, and their combinations. The model thus served to identify the most important gaps in our knowledge, and it specified the items of information which must be obtained if successful predictions were to be possible. Statistical extrapolation models can not perform this function.

Analogies with increased partnering activities associated with increased HPV transmission in recent years, and the consequent increase in cervical pathologies in young women, had already suggested in general and qualitative terms what the consequences might be for the spread of HIV. However, it was less clear, until the model was constructed and implemented, that a quantitative prediction required one other important parameter. This related to the age-correlation of those embarking upon new partnerships. With a chronic disease, the prevalence within a particular cohort increases as sexual experience widens. However, each new cohort, embarking on its own career pattern, could avoid much of the hazard if each individual stuck to his/her own age group, and did not mix with the highly infected cohorts already some years their senior. If, on the other hand, they are as indiscriminate about the ages of their partners as about their numbers, the infection will 'burn back' from the older to the younger age groups more rapidly than it is 'washed out' by aging from the top end of the age-distribution through diminishing participation or death.

If such a data requirement – emerging from a first model – is not appreciated and acted upon, then the design of sexual behaviour surveys intended to parametrise more advanced models, will be faulty. The moment of truth will arrive when these elaborated models are constructed and implemented. The data will be found to be deficient for the new purpose, and the prediction exercise will fail.

For reasons such as this the development of model systems and the design and implementation of sexual behaviour surveys must go hand in hand. Successive generations of models guide successive generations of field enquiry. Conversely, the difficulties and sometimes impracticabilities of certain field enquiries will restrain the rate and the manner in which the models are developed; and will restrict the questions that can be answered.

To sum up . . .

The AIDS emergency has stimulated an energetic and productive scientific response which has clarified the biology of the virus, its replication and its behaviour within human cells, the physical modes of its transmission and the pathogenesis of the consequent disease. However, scientific studies designed to support public health and preventive services have been far less incisive. A major emphasis has been placed upon statistical extrapolations, but these have been shown both in theory and in practice to be unreliable. They are also fundamentally incapable of evaluating proposed interventions.

Many epidemiological studies have been directed towards clarifying the internal biology of the disease process – measuring incubation periods, for example – but few have been directed towards an understanding of the population transmission processes and their control. These last issues can be guided only through the use of mechanistic transmission models based in turn upon measurements of contemporary sexual-social behaviours. Substantial developments in the representation of the mathematical relationships involved have been published, and several applications of these principles to sub-sections of populations have been implemented. Models representing multiple interacting behavioural groups have proved much more difficult because they demanded inputs of complex data which were simply not available. The need for such models, geared to local populations, remains. They offer the only route to rational planning, and there can be no such planning until this need is met. Our attempts to meet these needs are described in the next two sections of this book.

References

1. Shilts R. *And the Band Played On*. New York. 1987.

2. Knox E.G. (1986) 'A Transmission model for AIDS'. *Eur. J. Epid.* **2:** 165-177.

3. Kinsey A.C., Pomeroy W.B., Martin C.E. *Sexual Behaviour in the Human Male*. Philadelphia. 1948.

4. Knox E.G. (1984) 'Epidemic Cancer of the Cervix' In: *Hormones and sexual factors in human cancer aetiology*. Eds. J.P. Wolff and J.S. Scott. 125-138.

5. Knox E.G. and Shannon H.s. (1988) 'Cancer of the cervix and the papilloma viruses'. *Eur. J. Epid.* **1:** 83-92.

6. Biggar R.J., Bouvet E., Ebbesen P., Faber V., Koch M., Melbye M. and Velimirovic B. (1984) 'The Epidemiology of AIDS in Europe'. *Eur. J. Canc. Clin. Oncol.* **20:** 155-173.

7. PHLS Communicable Disease Surveillance Centre (1988) *Human Immunodeficiency Virus Infection in the United Kingdom: 2*. Communicable Disease Report. London.

8. Barre-Sinoussi F., Chermann J.C., Rey F et al. (1983) 'Isolation of T-lymphotropic retrovirus from a patient at risk for Acquired Immune Deficiency Syndrome (AIDS).' *Science* **220:** 868-870.

9. Gallo R.C., Salahuddin S.Z., Popovic M. et al. (1984) 'Frequent detection and isolation of cytopathic retroviruses (HTLV3) from patients with AIDS and at risk for AIDS.' *Science* **224:** 500-503.

10. Curran J.W., Morgan W.M., Hardy A.M., Jaffe H.W., Darrow W.W. and Dowdle W.R. (1985) 'The Epidemiology of AIDS: Current Status and Future Prospects'. *Science* **229:** 1352-1357.

11. Wong-Staal F. and Gallo R.C. (1985) 'Human T-lymphotropic retroviruses'. *Nature* **317:** 395-403.

12. Brandt A.M. (1988) 'AIDS in Historical Perspective: Four Lessons from the History of Sexually Transmitted Diseases'. *Amer. J. Pub. Hlth* **78:** 367-371.

13. Osborn J.E. (1989) 'AIDS and Public Policy'. *AIDS* **3:** 297-300.

14. Somerville M.A. and Orkin A.J. (1989) 'Human rights, discrimination and AIDS: concepts and issues'. *AIDS* **3:** 283-287.

15. Toomey K.E. and Cates Jr. W. (1989) 'Partner notification for the prevention of HIV infection'. *AIDS* **3:** 57-62.

16. Bayer R. (1989) 'Editorial review: Ethical and social policy issues raised by HIV screening: the epidemic evolves and so do the challenges'. *AIDS* **3:** 119-124.

17. British Medical Journal Legal Correspondent (1985) 'Detaining patients with AIDS'. *Brit. Med.J.* **291:** 1102.

18. Ohi G., Hasegawa T., Kai I., Inaba Y., Miyama T., Kamakura M., Terao H., Hirano W., Kobayashi Y., Muramatsu Y., Ashizawa M., Uemura I. and Niimi T. (1988) 'Notification of HIV carriers: Possible effect on uptake of AIDS testing'. *Lancet* **2:** 947-949.

19. WHO (1988) *Avoidance of discrimination in relation to HIV infected people and people with AIDS.* Resolution of the 41st World Assembly in Geneva.

20. Committee of Ministers: Council of Europe (1987) *Concerning a common European public health policy to fight the Acquired Immunodeficiency Syndrome (AIDS).* Recommendation No. R (87) 25.

21. General Medical Council (1988) *HIV infection and AIDS: The ethical considerations.*

22. Council of Europe Committee of Ministers. (1990) *The ethical issues of HIV infection in the health care and social settings.* Recommendation No. R (89) 14.

23. Acheson, Sir Donald (1988) *A Report of the Committee of Inquiry into the Future Development of the Public Health Function.* HMSO. London.

24. Brookmeyer R. and Damiano A. (1989) 'Statistical Methods for Short-Term Projections of AIDS Incidence'. *Statistics in Medicine* **8:** 23-34.

25. Taylor J.M.G., Schwartz K. and Detels R. (1986) 'The Time from Infection with Human Immunodeficiency Virus (HIV) to the Onset of AIDS'. *J. Infect. Dis.* **154:** 694-697.

26. Lui K.J, Lawrence D.N., Morgan W.M., Peterman T.A., Haverkos H.W. and Bregman D.J. (1986) 'A model-based approach for estimating the mean incubation period of transfusion-associated acquired immunodeficiency syndrome'. *Proc. Nat. Acad. Sci.* **83:**

27. Bacchetti P. and Moss A.R. (1989) 'Incubation period of AIDS in San Francisco'. *Nature* **338:** 251-253.

28. Lagakos S.W., Barraj L.M. and Gruttola V. (1988) 'Nonparametric analysis of truncated survival data, with application to AIDS'. *Biometrika* **75:** 515-23.

29. Munoz A., Wang M.C., Bass S., Taylor J.M.G., Kingsley L.A., Chmiel J.S., Polk B.F. and The Multicenter AIDS Cohort Study Group. (1989) 'Acquired Immunodeficiency Syndrome (AIDS)-Free Time After Human Immunodeficiency Virus Type 1 (HIV-1) Seroconversion in Homosexual Men'. *Amer. J. Epidem.* **130:** 530-539.

30. Brookmeyer R. and Goedert J.J. (1989) 'Censoring in an Epidemic with an Application to Hemophilia-Associated AIDS'. *Biometrics* **45:** 325-335.

31. Cox D. (1987) 'Estimation of the incubation period' In: *Future Trends in AIDS: A Seminar to discuss the prediction of the AIDS Epidemic.* HMSO, London. 1987.

32. Downs A.M., Ancelle R.A., Jager J.C., Heisterkamp S.H., van Druten J.A.M., Ruitenberg E.J. and Brunet J.B. (1988) 'The statistical estimation, from routine surveillance data, of past, present, and future trends in AIDS incidence in Europe'. In: *Statistical Analysis and Mathematical Modelling of AIDS.* Eds. J.C. Jager and E.J. Ruitenberg. New York 1988.

33. Heisterkamp S.H., Jager J.C., Downs A.M., van Druten J.A.M., and Ruitenberg E.J. (1988) 'Statistical estimation of AIDS incidence from surveillance data and the link with modelling of trends'. In: *Statistical Analysis and Mathematical Modelling of AIDS.* Eds. J.C. Jager and E.J. Ruitenberg. New York 1988.

34. Richardson, S.C., Caroni C. and Papaevangelou G. (1988) 'Predicting the AIDS epidemic from trends elsewhere'. In: *Statistical Analysis and Mathematical Modelling of AIDS.* Eds. J.C. Jager and E.J. Ruitenberg. New York 1988.

35. Pickering J., Wiley J.A., Lieb L.E., Walker J. and Rutherford G.W. 'Modelling the Incidence of AIDS in New York, Los Angeles and San Francisco'. In: *Statistical Analysis and Mathematical Modelling of AIDS.* Eds. J.C. Jager and E.J. Ruitenberg. New York 1988.

36. Healy M.J.R. and Tillett H.E. (1988) 'Short-term Extrapolation of the AIDS Epidemic'. *J.R. Statist. Soc.* **151:** 50-65.

37. Day N.E., Gore S.M., McGee M.A. and South M. (1989) 'Predictions of the AIDS epidemic in the U.K.: The use of the Back Projection Method'. *Phil. Trans. R. Soc. Lond.* **325:** 123-134.

38. Isham V. (1989) 'Estimation of the Incidence of HIV Infection'. *Phil. Trans. R. Soc. Lond.* **325:** 113-121.

39. Day N.E. (Chairman) (1990) 'Acquired Immune Deficiency Syndrome in England and Wales to End 1993: Projections Using Data to End September 1989. *PHLS. CDR.* 41: 195.

40. Ala F., Smyllie J., Nicholson G., Gough D., Duddin R. and Knox E.G. (1991) 'Unlinked Surveillance of the Prevalence of HIV Infection in antenatal patients in the West Midlands, England'. *J. Med. Virol.* **34:** 176-178.

41. Banatvala J.E., Chrystie I.L., Palmer S.J., Sumner D., Kennedy J., Kenney A. (1991) 'HIV screening in pregnancy'. *Lancet* **337:** 12-18.

42. Koch M.G. (1991) *Pathogenesis of AIDS and the Logics of a Tardive Epidemic: Why is HIV so Malevolently Successful?.* Presentation to British Society of Haematology: Glasgow.

43. En'ko P.D. (1889) 'The epidemic course of some infectious diseases'. *Vrac* **10**, 1008-1010, 1039-1042, 1061-1063.

44. Hamer W.H. (1906) 'Epidemic disease in England – the evidence of variability and of persistency of type. *Lancet ii.* 733-739.

45. Ross R. *Report on the Prevention of Malaria in Mauritius.* London 1908.

46. Ross R. *The Prevention of Malaria.* London 1911.

47. Fine P.E.M. (1979) 'John Brownlee and the Measurement of Infectiousness: An Historical Study in Epidemic Theory'. *J.R.Statist.Soc.* Series A **142:** 347-362.

48. van Druten J.A.M. *A Mathematical-Statistical Model for the Analysis of Cross-Sectional Serological Data with special reference to the Epidemiology of Malaria.* Katholieke Universiteit Nijmegan. 1981.

49. Bailey N.T.J. *The Mathematical Theory of Epidemics.* London: 1957.

50. Bailey N.T.J. and Thomas, Anthony S. (1971) 'The Estimation of Parameters from Population Data on the General Stochastic Epidemic'. *Theoret. Popul. Biology* **2:** 253-270.

51. Elveback L. and Varma A. (1965) 'Simulation of Mathematical Models for Public Health Problems'. *Publ. Hlth. Reports* **80:** 1067-1076.

52. De Velle, Charles S., Lynn, Walter R., and Feldmann Floyd (1967) 'Mathematical Models for the Economic Allocation of Tuberculosis Control Activities in Developing Nations.' *Amer. Rev. Resp. Dis.* **96:** 893-909.

53. Gatewood L.C., Ackerman E., Ewy W., Elveback L. and Fox J.P. (1971) 'Simulation of Models of Enteric Virus Epidemics'. *Medical Computing* **2:** 201-213.

54. Cvjetanovic B., Grab B. and Uemura K. (1971) 'Epidemiological Model of Typhoid Fever and its Use in the Planning and Evaluation of Antityphoid Immuniza-tion and Sanitation Programmes' *Bull. Wld. Hlth. Org.* **45:** 53-75.

55. Cvjetanovic B., Grab B. and Uemura K. (1978) 'Dynamics of Acute Bacterial Diseases'. Supplement No. 1 to Vol. **56** of *Bulletin* of *WHO*.

56. Elveback L.R., Fox J.P., Ackerman E., Langworthy A., Boyd M. and Gatewood L. (1976) 'An Influenza Simulation Model for Immunization Studies'. *Amer. J. Epidem.* **103:** 152-165.

57. Bartoszynski R. (1975) 'A Model for Risk of Rabies'. In: *Proceedings of the 40th Session.* Bulletin of the International Statistical Institute. Warsaw.

58. Ackerman E., Elveback L.R. and Fox J.P. *Simulation of Infectious Diseases.* Illinois 1984.

59. Zhang Yangzi (1987) 'A Compound Catalytic Model with both Reversible and Two-Stage Types and its Applications in Epidemiological Study'. *Int.J. Epidem.* **16:** 619-621.

60. Dietz, K. (1967) 'Epidemics and Rumors: A survey'. *J.R.Statist. Soc.* Series A. **130:** 505-528.

61. Dietz. K. (1975) 'Models for Parasitic Disease Control'. In: *Proceedings of the 40th Session.* Bulletin of the International Statistical Institute. Warsaw.

62. Anderson R.M. and May R.M. (Eds.) *Population Biology of Infectious Diseases.* Report of the Dahlem Workshop on Population Biology of Infectious Disease Agents. Berlin. 1982.

63. Anderson R.M. (1982) 'Transmission Dynamics and Control of Infectious Disease Agents'. In *Population Biology of Infectious Diseases,* eds. Anderson and May. 149-176.

64. Knox E.G. (1980) 'Strategy for Rubella Vaccination'. *Int. J. Epidem.* **9:** 13-23.

65. Knox E.G. (1987) 'Evolution of Rubella Vaccine Policy for the U.K.'. *Int. J. Epidem.* **16:** 569-578.

66. Anderson R.M. and Grenfell B.T. (1986) 'Quantitative investigations of different vaccination policies for the control of congenital rubella syndrome (CRS) in the United Kingdom'. *J. Hyg.* **96:** 305-333.

67. May R.M. and Anderson R.M. (1984) 'Spatial Heterogeneity and the Design of Immunization Programs'. *Mathematical Biosciences* **72:** 83-111.

68. Katzmann W. and Dietz K. (1984) 'Evaluation of Age-Specific Vaccination Strategies'. *Theoretical Population Biology* **25:** 125-137.

69. Knox E.G. and Shannon H.S. (1986) 'A Model Basis for the Control of Whooping Cough' *Int. J. Epidem.* **15:** 544-552.

70. Cvjetanovic B., Grab B., Uemura K. and Bytchenko B. (1972) 'Epidemiological Model of Tetanus and its Use in the Planning of Immunization Programmes'. *Int. J. Epidem.* **1:** 125-137.

71. Knox E.G. (1976) 'Ages and Frequencies for Cervical Cancer Screening'. *Br. J. Cancer* **34:** 444-452.

72. Knox E.G. (1973) 'Computer simulations of cervical cytology screening programmes'. In: *Future and present indicatives, Problems and Progress in Medical Care.* 9th Series. Ed. G. McLachlan. Published for Nuffield Provincial Hospitals Trust, London, Oxford University Press. 30-55.

73. Knox E.G. (1975) 'Simulation Studies of Breast Cancer Screening Programmes'. In: *Probes for Health.* Ed. G. McLachlan. Published for Nuffield Provincial Hospitals Trust, London, Oxford University Press, 14-44.

74. Constable G.M. (1975) 'The problems of V.D. Modelling'. In: *Proceedings of the 40th Session.* Bulletin of the International Statistical Institute. Warsaw.

75. Reynolds G.H. and Chan Yick-Kwong (1975) 'A control model for gonorrhoea'. In: *Proceedings of the 40th Session.* Bulletin of the International Statistical Institute. Warsaw.

76. Yorke J.A., Hethcote H.W. and Nold A. (1978) 'Dynamics and Control of the Transmission of Gonorrhea'. *Sexually Transmitted Diseases.* **5:** 51-56.

77. Lajmanovich X. and Yorke J.A. (1976) 'A Deterministic Model for Gonorrhea in a Nonhomogeneous Population'. *Mathematical Biosciences* **28:** 221-236.

78. Heisterkamp S.H., De Haan B.J., Jager J.C., Van Druten J.A.M. and Hendriks J.C.M. (1992) 'Short and medium term Projections of the AIDS/HIV Epidemic by a dynamic model with an application to the risk group of Homo/Bisexual men in Amsterdam'. *Statistics in Medicine* **11:** 1425-1441

79. Stigum H., Gronnesby J.K., Magnus P., Sundet J.M. and Bakketeig L.S. (1991) 'The Potential for spread of HIV in the Heterosexual Population in Norway: A Model Study'. *Statistics in Medicine* **10:** 1003-1023.

80. May R.M. and Anderson R.M. (1987) 'Transmission dynamics of HIV infection'. *Nature* **326:** 137-142.

81. Anderson R.M. (1988) 'The Epidemiology of HIV Infection: Variable Incubation Plus Infectious Periods and Heterogeneity in Sexual Activity'. *J.R. Statist. Soc.* **151:** 66-98.

82. Jacquez J.A., Simon C.P., Koopman J., Sattenspiel L. and Perry T. (1988) ' Modeling and Analyzing HIV Transmission: The Effect of Contact Patterns'. *Mathematical Biosciences* **92:** 119-199.

83. Kaplan E.H. (1989) 'Can Bad Models Suggest Good Policies? Sexual Mixing and the AIDS Epidemic'. *The Journal of Sex Research* **26:** 301-314.

84. Kaplan E.H. and Lee Y.S. (1989) 'How bad can it get? Bounding Worst Case Endemic Heterogeneous Mixing Models of HIV/AIDS'. *Mathematical Biosciences* **99:** 157-180.

85. Doust J.A. 1990) 'Annotated Bibliography' In: *Projections of Acquired Immune Deficiency Syndrome in Australia using data to the end of September 1989.* National Centre for Epidemiology and Population Health, The Australian National University.

86. Van Druten J.A.M., Reintjes A.G.M., Jager J.C., Heisterkamp S.H., Poos M.J.J.C., Coutinho R.A., Dijkgraaf M.G.W. and Ruitenberg E.J. (1990) 'HIV Infection Dynamics and Intervention Experiments in Linked Risk Groups'. *Statistics in Medicine* **9:** 721-736.

PART TWO

Sexual Behaviour in Britain

Chapter 6 – Design and Rationale of a Sexual Behaviour Survey

Part Two of this report describes the purposes, the design, the sampling base, the methods, and the results, of a survey of sexual behaviour in the West Midlands Region of England. The survey-method was developed through a series of stages and the final design was decided after extensive piloting. The choice was conditioned by a number of prior social, technical and financial constraints, including the available time and staff resources, while others were imposed later by contingencies encountered during the course of the investigation.

The purposes of the sexual behaviour survey were quite closely defined. They were to provide sexual behaviour data sufficient to inform a predictive simulation model which had been designed to mimic HIV transmission within a heterogeneous population; and particularly data regarding those sexual events and circumstances which would facilitate or hinder the growth of the epidemic or modify its character. These data requirements had been clarified at an earlier stage through the development of a simple epidemic model, designed to predict an eventual equilibrium position (1, 2). However, the data requirements were progressively enlarged and refined as a more complex and discriminating model was developed. Much additional information would be needed in order to mimic the detailed dynamics of epidemic growth over a period of many years, in many different sub-sections of the population: as well as in the population as a whole.

The construction of the new model and the development of the survey technique were conducted simultaneously and each process made demands or imposed constraints upon the other. By the time that both were finalised, the model had passed through three separate stages of structuring and re-structuring, with two phases of development of the input parameters. These processes were conditioned by the availability of particular items of data, as revealed in pilot field surveys, but technical constraints continued to appear throughout the whole of the development. Even during the 'production runs' of the model, as the results were obtained, we found that we had to 'trim' the parameters repeatedly, and even introduce new ones, before we had a practical predictive tool.

The survey was designed to provide a quantitative description of heterosexual, homosexual and mixed homosexual/heterosexual behaviour in the general population; and to show the ways in which these behaviour patterns varied between different age groups, by gender, between different ethnic groups, different social groups, different educational groups and different birth cohorts. And to measure the degree of variation *within* these groups. The essential descriptor of sexual behaviour variations – as required by the model – was the 'rate of acquisition of new sexual partners'. This concept had been developed earlier, during the construction of a model of Human Papilloma Virus (HPV) transmission in relation to cervical cancer (3, 4) and used subsequently in our HIV equilibrium model (1).

A parameter thus defined is not one which a respondent answering a questionnaire might readily grasp. Even in a face-to-face interview it is not a satisfactory subject for a direct question. In any case, it is an inconstant parameter which changes at successive ages and at different stages of a sexual career. For partners after the first partner it amounts to the reciprocal of the mean interval between the establishment of new partnerships; but there would be great problems, still, in posing a question in these terms. In practice, it requires the identification of each separate partnership by each respondent, together with a statement of the respondent's and the partner's ages at the time, the calendar year in which the partnership was established, and its duration. In the event, the complexity of some of the sexual histories made full and accurate ascertainment impossible.

At any given point in time – both in real life and within a representative model – the next increment of the HIV epidemic depends simultaneously upon the current values for four main parameters. As well as the rate of acquisition of new partners (above) the additional determinants are i) the durations of these partnerships, ii) the current proportions of susceptibles and infecteds within the population, and iii) the risk of infective transmission per unit time during the course of any partnership in which one member is infective (HIV positive) and the other susceptible (HIV negative).

The parameter values differ in different sub-strata of the population, and the epidemic course is different within each of them: but not independently so, because of contacts between the different age-bands and cohorts, and between different sexual behaviour groups with varying sexual preferences and varying frequencies of partner acquisition. The risk of transmission also varies between different forms of sexual contact. For example, the risk of transmission from males to females is different from the risk of transmission from females to males; and transmission from a penetrative to a receptive male homosexual differs from the reverse risk. Even within particular behaviour classes, the frequency of sexual intercourse varies widely and with it, presumably, the risk of transmission per unit time.

The possibility of reaching a finite equilibrium within any sub-stratum depends upon the combination of parameters encountered. In a behaviourally heterogeneous hetero-sexual population, consisting of many mutually isolated sub-groups, the infection could survive in some of these groups but not in others. However, because the separate strata are in practice not totally isolated , there will be a continuing quasi-equilibrium based upon continual 'seeding' from the intrinsically self-maintaining strata, to the others. For example, the groups of heterosexual males and females who change partners at the modest rates defined later as 'level-1', may not achieve a sufficient flow of infection between them to maintain an equilibrium; yet both may be sufficiently 'seeded' through contacts with individuals following more intensive (level-2 or level-3) activity patterns, to maintain a steady prevalence. An understanding of the pattern of behavioural heterogeneity is therefore essential to an understanding of the epidemic itself.

Our previous model (1) had already shown that the heterosexual component of the epidemic was likely in the long run to be the largest component, outstripping the homosexual and drug-using components, provided that it turned out to be self-sustaining. The main long-term role of the smaller high risk groups would then be to facilitate the social and geographical spread of the disease and to 'seed' the heterosexuals. Heterosexual self-sustenance might also be limited to only a part of the heterosexual population which would itself 'seed' the remainder.

The question of self-sustenance, and its extent, is also critical for designing policies for containing the epidemic. If the disease were not self-sustaining within any of the heterosexual groups, then preventive measures could be concentrated upon high risk groups – promiscuous homosexuals, intravenous drug-users, and perhaps heterosexuals with other sexually transmitted diseases (STD). On the other hand, if heterosexual spread were likely to be self-sustaining, – even if limited to a core group as in the case of gonorrhoea – then a more widely directed preventive process would be required.

Ancillary Enquiries

Although our primary concern in the survey was with the statistical and demographic distributions of rates of partner switching among our respondents, two other requirements emerged from the initial modelling exercise. First, we needed information on the characteristics of the sexual partners of the respondents, as well as the respondents themselves. Second, we needed information on behavioural idiosyncrasies which might influence the risk of virus transmission from an infected to a susceptible partner. The first of these needs related chiefly to the ages of the partners, and the second to variations in sexual practices, including the monthly frequency of sexual intercourse, the use of condoms, the proportions engaging in heterosexual anal intercourse, and other indicators of higher risk sexual behaviour such as a history of STD.

We needed to know about the ages of partners because the prevalence of a chronic (long-lasting) infection increases with age, and different partner age-preferences expose the seeker to different risks. A high rate of infection in young susceptibles depends upon contacts with partners of greater ages. The rate of spread depends upon whether people from low prevalence and high prevalence age-groups contact only partners with the same prevalence level; or whether, more dangerously, their contacts cross the boundary between the high prevalence and low prevalence components of the population. The balance between dispersion and concentration is important, and this extends to factors other than age, including sexual style, and social and geographical isolation. A sufficient degree of concentration and group-isolation is necessary in order to generate a self-sustaining process; and yet a sufficient dispersion of contact is necessary if the epidemic is to reach a substantial proportion of the population.

These issues were complicated by the cohort variations in sexual behaviour which we found. For example, when we tried to demonstrate the growth of prevalence with age by displaying cumulative numbers of partners reported by respondents in different age bands, we found that the 'curve of accumulation' appeared in some groups to have gone into reverse. Our sample seemed to have achieved the impossible in having accumulated more partners by age 25 than by age 45. This was of course a cohort effect, rather than a true accumulation of partners; the recent cohorts had already overtaken those cohorts born ten or twenty years earlier.

For the men, we wanted to know whether and how often they had used the services of female prostitutes. We also asked the men about the use of male homosexual prostitutes for anal intercourse.

The risk of transmission within those partnerships where one member is infective depends ultimately upon the duration of the partnership, the frequency of intercourse within the partnership, and the risk of transmission per individual contact. In practical terms, the last value is not directly measurable on an event-observation basis, and it has to be derived indirectly from observations of sero-conversion rates and of intercourse rates per unit time. Partly for this reason, some authors have concatenated these elements in various ways, devising such terms as 'effective contact' (5), or have expressed the risk on a 'per partnership' basis (1, 6, 7, 8). In the present exercise we have adopted a time-based expression of risk. In methodological terms, ultimate 'per contact' values are derived from observations of change over measured periods of time and we found it easier, and indeed more legitimate, to work directly in terms of rates of change per unit time – rather than from retrospectively back-calculated 'per contact' values. This is the approach adopted here.

There is one additional way, apart from direct sexual contacts between members of different behavioural groups, in which the prevalence of an infection may diffuse from one sub-group to another. Persons within one sub group may themselves move to another through changing their behaviour, thus transferring a fraction of the prevalence in their first sub-group, to the second one. The first mechanism is through demographic transfers such as marriage and divorce. For example, a bi-sexual or homosexual single male may marry and adopt a purely heterosexual behaviour pattern. The transfer of infection from one sub-group to another through this mechanism turns out to be an important transfer pathway (see later), and one which has been noted by other workers. Bi-sexual or homosexual males may revert to purely heterosexual behaviour in the absence of marriage: or vice versa. A woman may switch from a promiscuous single to a prostitute; and a single prostitute may marry and may either give up or retain her profession. We therefore asked about heterosexual and about male homosexual contacts – the important ones from our point of view – in such a way as to construct a picture of sexual career patterns among current heterosexuals and homosexuals; and among people with mixed experiences, whether parallel or serial.

Finally, we would ideally wish to know, for persons with different levels of partner-acquisition, what were the acquisition levels among their contacts. We could not carry out such an enquiry within the format of our study, but the effect of an activity correlation such as this would be that the partners of highly-active high-prevalence sub-groups would themselves be highly active: and also have relatively high prevalences of HIV infectivity. The effect would be to create 'core group' concentrations of activity and infectivity, a contingency with exactly the opposite effect of career-shift diffusion (above). Our information on these two opposing phenomena were so deficient as to bar their direct utilisation within the model. Their effects are nevertheless sufficiently important to require that they be taken into account. We shall describe an indirect approach to the representation of these phenomena in a later part of this monograph.

Restrictions and Limitations

The method of data-assembly which we eventually adopted – a self-completed questionnaire-form presented during a short break at the place of work – effectively restricted the number of questions we could ask. We therefore decided *not* to collect information on matters tangential to our primary objectives. We did not ask for information on knowledge or attitudes regarding the sexual transmission of infections or of HIV in particular. The method was also unsuitable for collecting information on particular sexual practices apart from simple factual questions concerning homosexual and heterosexual anal intercourse, the 'usual' frequency of sexual intercourse, and the use of condoms. We did not extend this enquiry to the question of oral intercourse. We did not ask about drug addiction or needle sharing and we did not ask about relatives or contacts with HIV or other STD's. Female homosexual relationships were not asked about either, because of their lack of relevance for HIV transmission. Finally, we had to work within a commitment to anonymity which barred the possibility of measuring changes over time in individuals – because they could not be contacted again. The need for visible anonymity also restricted the specificity of some of our questions, particularly with respect to exact ages and exact dates, which were in general limited to formats expressed in whole years. It also barred the possibility of validating reports through interviewing a sub-sample, or asking supplementary questions, or repeating the questionnaire.

Sample Checks

We did however, enquire into certain items which would help us characterise the sample, to compare it with the general population, and to estimate the level of discrepancies between the two. To this end we enquired about ethnic group, age, sex and birth cohort, occupation, marital status, age at leaving full-time education, educational qualifications, number of children, whether and how often they had suffered from a sexually transmitted disease and (for women) how many pregnancy terminations they had had.

Finally, we used a confidential serial number to tag the source-Institution – to which we guaranteed anonymity – within which the data collection had taken place. In most instances this was the place of work itself: but for those 'on release' for technical training or further education, we used the place of data assembly. To each source we attached a 'response rate': i.e. the proportion of eligible persons who completed the questionnaire. From this, and by comparing similar institutions with different response-levels, we hoped to obtain an indication of the level of bias – in terms of sexual activity levels – which respondent self-selection might incur.

Chapter 7 – Method of Enquiry

We did not know, at first, what level of return we would obtain from alternative sampling frames and alternative approaches: whether in terms of response rates, the accuracy of the replies, or the representative nature of the results. We knew only that we would have to accept some kind of compromise and that there was no way of reconciling the need for a socially representative sample, with a response sufficiently high to eliminate the dangers of responder bias; or of reconciling a desirable level of detail with the numbers required and the available research resources, and with the willingness of our respondents to assist. There was also a danger, with such a sensitive subject, that any false steps or unfavourable publicity might prevent us from completing the job. We therefore developed our methods in a very cautious manner, avoiding all contact with the media, and the investigation went through a large series of pilot investigations before we settled on its final form. Originally, we thought we would have to use face-to-face questioning, the interviewer completing the first part of a structured form to collect basic demographic data (age, sex, marital status etc.), and the respondent completing the more sensitive questions in private. An approach where all the information was collected in a face-to-face contact was not considered suitable because of the likelihood of limited acceptance, and of reticent or untruthful answers in a situation where individuals might feel embarrassed, or that they might be identified. As we began to pilot the enquiry, however, we were steered down other pathways.

In the early pilots, where we explored a variety of different techniques, our respondents expressed a firm preference for the private self-completion of the whole of an anonymous questionnaire. They did not want to be interviewed or personally instructed or assisted. It also became clear that it was both possible and preferable for them to 'fill in' a self-completed questionnaire in groups under the general supervision of the investigators. This could be preceded by a careful initial explanation to the whole group from a member of the research team, the completion of the enquiry-form then taking place under 'examination room' conditions. The respondents, or more accurately their employers, were willing to spend thirty minutes on the task, but not much more. In many circumstances it was much more convenient for staff to be released in groups and return to work together: rather than be released separately. In some cases they completed their forms at the work 'bench'. There was also considerable economy, for the researchers as well as the institutions, if respondents could be handled in groups of 10 to 30, rather than singly as was our initial plan.

The piloting was conducted using a variety of 'work' groups and included manual, clerical and professional workers. However we specifically concentrated on employees with lower educational levels who would be unfamiliar with written work and form-filling. This was in order to develop a questionnaire that would be understood by the majority of literate individuals. In all the pilot investigations the respondents were

37

interviewed afterwards, to comment upon their understanding of the questions, and to offer suggestions for their improvement. Reports completed during the pilot investigations were not used in the main analyses.

It was anticipated that these pilot groups would not contain enough homosexual men to develop and pilot the relevant questions adequately, for this group. Special pilot investigations of larger groups of homosexual men were therefore arranged on our behalf, recruiting them within various gay venues. Like the other pilot groups, they completed the pilot questionnaires and then discussed and commented afterwards on their understanding and the appropriateness of the questions.

We discovered that the 'group ethos' of questionnaire-completion resulted in a bimodal pattern of response in different institutions; either we could gain no access at all: or else near-total access. In favourable circumstances we reached upwards of 90 percent of the individuals on the premises at the time. We could also keep a running note of the percentage response at each location; and, later on, try to assess the effects of different response rates and of potential response-bias upon our results.

Accuracy and Validity

The modified format of enquiry had several secondary effects. First, because there was no prompting or secondary questioning, it was not possible to correct ambiguities, or check whether each respondent had properly understood each question. We therefore built into the questionnaire a series of redundancies and cross-checks to assess the consistency of different answers; and sometimes diagnose the nature of the errors or inconsistencies. This stage of development took longer than anticipated and the process went through many pilots before we were reasonably satisfied with the results.

The limitations of accuracy and detail intrinsic to a questionnaire suited to a maximum of twenty minutes for its completion, appeared in the course of analysis. Although the questionnaires were completed in a sensible manner by the respondents, substantial numbers found ways of misunderstanding or misinterpreting some of the questions. It would have been possible to counter some of these misinterpretations through appending extra clauses to the questions or additional explanatory notes in the introduction, but we found in our pilot studies that if the questions were elaborated so as to be universally and logically explicit – like legal documents – then they were likely to be understood by no one. The final version sought a compromise between the risk of the two kinds of misunderstanding.

We found little guidance in the literature regarding the relative merits of face-to-face and group methods in sexual behaviour enquiries. There are several reported studies comparing personal interviews with other forms of enquiry (9) but we found little to guide us with respect to the technique which we eventually adopted. It is largely for these reasons that we spent so much time at the pilot stage, seeking responses to repeated reformulations and using our respondents' views to guide us.

Working Practices

The questionnaire sessions were always preceded by a formal introduction by a member of the research team who adopted a serious approach to the topic which in turn engendered a like approach on the part of the respondents. The group were thanked for their participation, and the researcher explained broadly what the study was for. Emphasis was placed on the anonymous nature of the questionnaire. Particular points of difficulty or possible misunderstanding were explained and the respondents were then invited to fill in the questions one after the other, taking care not to write down anything which they felt might compromise their anonymity. That is, if their exact occupations might identify them within the particular context, or the combination of their age, their sex and their ethnic group (say), then they were invited to omit answering one of the questions. They were invited simply to skip any questions to which they objected – although in practice very few did so. They were also explicitly told at this stage that anyone who wished could leave; or if they wanted to opt out 'in private' they could stay but not complete the questionnaire. It was very rare for anyone to walk out, but there were a few who left blank questionnaires. The latter were then counted among the non-responders.

The forms themselves were carefully structured, and the first piloted versions had contained written instructions to skip certain sections if – on the basis of an earlier question – they were irrelevant. In our piloting experience with these forms however we found that we had to restructure them so that it would not be possible from one part of the room to be able to tell whether another respondent was spending a greater or lesser amount of time on a particular section by observing the manner in which he/she turned the pages. In our final questionnaire design, all respondents had to answer all questions, with the exception of those who had had no sexual experience. The respondents were asked to stay to the end of the defined period, even though they might have already completed their forms; and all were asked to finish after twenty minutes, even if they had not yet completed them. This was in order to avoid possible comments from colleagues of the time taken by particular individuals to write everything down, with corresponding implications regarding the number of partners they had to remember. In the piloting stages it was observed that after about twenty minutes almost everyone had finished, and those who had not were unable to improve on what they had already written. Occasionally, if a group was well used to form-filling, the time allocation was reduced to fifteen minutes. In the early stages we discovered that we sometimes had to operate under rather crowded conditions, for example in a staff room or on a laboratory bench. We therefore had specially made for us portable screens consisting of three pieces of plywood connected with piano hinges, which could be stood on any work surface around the respondent's form. These were always given out, although respondents occasionally chose not to put up their screen. At the end of the session the respondents all sealed their forms into unmarked envelopes and dropped them into a padlocked 'ballot box'.

The questions on the questionnaire forms are provided in Appendix A7 (although not in the actual page format) together with an outline introduction from which individual oral presentations were given.

APPENDIX 7

Introduction to Sexual Behaviour Questionnaire

All of the following points should be included in the introductory talk.

My name is .... and I am part of a team from the Medical School at the University who are carrying out a very large study for the Medical Research Council in London. It is a very important study which has the aim of finding out more about how HIV and AIDS might spread. Hundreds of people will eventually be included in the study.

At the moment in this country the number of people with the AIDS virus is not huge. You probably don't know many people, if any, who have it. Gradually more and more people will get HIV and AIDS. We know that it is going to spread. However, what we don't know is how quickly it will spread or how best to stop it. To be able to predict this, we urgently need to know more about the sexual behaviour of people in this country, since this is how the virus is spread. That is what this study is about.

It is necessary to be able to predict the spread of AIDS for several reasons. We have to plan the health services that will be needed by people with the disease. We need to know which groups will have to have intensive health education programmes. And when a vaccine becomes available we need to know which groups to give it to.

When the information on sexual behaviour has been collected it will be entered into a computer and predictions can be made about the spread of AIDS.

We are here today to ask if you will take part in this study. I will tell you more about it first. We must stress that all the information you give us will be anonymous and confidential. There are no names or other way of identifying individuals on the questionnaire. Once you have sealed your finished questionnaire in the envelope and put it into the box, no one will know who has answered it. They are not opened until all those from this institution have been completed. We will never have any way of knowing who filled in which questionnaire.

So that we can know how our sample compares with people in this country we ask questions about age, family circumstances, ethnic group and occupation. These questions are on the first page. If however you feel that any of your answers will identify you, just miss them out. On the last page of the questionnaire we ask other questions, again for similar reasons.

We want to include in the study people who have had no sexual partners and people who have had many. All of the other questions are about your sexual partners. By this we don't just mean wives/husbands and girlfriends/boyfriends, but everyone you have had sexual intercourse with, including one night stands and other casual partners. We are asking about your whole life, so some things may be difficult to remember. You will have more than enough time to finish, so take as much time as your need. Please be as accurate as you can and try to check your answers.

There are some questions which have given people trouble in the past, and it might be useful to tell you a little more about these questions before you answer them.

The first is **QUESTION 12**. *(All have questionnaires to look at)*. This question is about the last ten men/women you had sexual intercourse with. We would like to stress that this means absolutely everybody, however long ago this was, and however short the sexual relationship was. If you can't remember all the details about every single one, for example how old the person was, please just put in the question that there was a person.

Next, **QUESTION 13**, over the page. This is about the number of **new** sexual partners in each of the last six years. By **new** sexual partner we mean somebody whom you have not had sexual intercourse with before. We find that it is helpful here if we give examples to make this clear. *(Give detailed examples using names, dates, etc., stressing again what new partners is and showing how boxes would be filled in)*.

QUESTION 14 is similar, except that it covers your whole life, so all your sexual partners will be counted here. This question asks how old you were when you had each **new** sexual partner. *(Examples again)*.

We ask people to fill in the questionnaire without talking, i.e. under 'exam conditions'. We will give you 20 minutes to fill in the questionnaire which will be plenty of time. When you have finished please would you stay in your seat without moving the screens until we ask you to stop and 'post' the sealed questionnaire.

If anyone doesn't want to take part in the survey either they can leave the room or stay and just leave the form blank. However, we would like to stress again how serious and important the study is, that it is completely anonymous, and that we would be extremely grateful to everyone who does take part.

We would be very happy to answer any questions about the study when the questionnaires have been completed.

Questionnaire for Women

1. What is your year of birth? . . . .

2. What is your job? . . . .
   If you are married, what is your husband's job? . . . .

3. How old were you when you left school/fulltime education? ☐

4. Did you get any qualifications and if so what? . . . .
   . . . .

5. What is your present marital status? *(Tick one)*

   | Single | ☐ | Divorced | ☐ | Widowed | ☐ |
   | Married | ☐ | Separated | ☐ | | |

6. Who do you live with? *(Tick more than one if necessary)*

   | Alone | ☐ | Husband | ☐ | Friend(s) | ☐ |
   | Parent(s) | ☐ | Partner | ☐ | Other | ☐ |

7. Would you please answer some questions about any **marriages**, and **partners you have lived with**?

	What year did you start living with your husband or partner?	How long did you live with your husband or partner?	Did you marry?
Husband or Partner 1			
" " " 2			
" " " 3			
" " " 4			
" " " 5			
" " " 6			

8. How many children have you? ☐

43

9. What is your ethnic group?

European/White ☐   Indian/Pakistani/Bangladeshi ☐

African/Afro-Caribbean ☐   Other ☐

First we would like to ask you about your sexual experiences with men

10. Have you ever had sexual intercourse with a man?

Yes ☐   No ☐

If the answer is 'NO' do not answer any more questions

11. How old were you when you first had intercourse? ☐

12. These questions are about the **last ten women** you have had sexual intercourse with.

Include one night stands, casual and longer-term partners

For each woman please fill in all of the boxes. Start with the woman you have most recently had sexual intercourse with.

	What year did you first have sexual intercourse with him?	Do you still have intercourse with her? *YES/NO*	If *NO*, how long did this sexual relationship last?	About how old was the man at the start?	About how often do/did you have intercourse each month on average?	Do/did you use condoms *(ALWAYS, USUALLY, SOMETIMES, NEVER)*
Most recent						
One before						
One before						
One before						
One before						
One before						
One before						
One before						
One before						
One before						

*The questions which follow on the next pages may seem similar and for some people the answers may be almost the same. They are however slightly different, in ways which can be important. Would you therefore please try to **answer them all** as carefully as you can?*

13. *How many* **new** *sexual partners have you had in each of the* **last six years**?

Include one night stands, casual and longer-term partners

Year

1991	
1990	Place a Number or (0)
1989	in each box
1988	
1987	
1986	

14. People often have different numbers of sexual relationships during different ages in their life. We need to find out about this.

How many **new** sexual partners did you have when you were aged:–

Include one night stands, casual and longer-term partners

17 yrs or less	
18-19 years	
20-24 years	
25-29 years	*Place a Number or (0)*
30-34 years	*in each box up to your*
35-39 years	*present age*
40-44 years	
45-49 years	
50 yrs or more	

15. About how many men have you had intercourse with **in your life**? *(Please ring whichever number is applicable)*

1 2 3 4 5 6 7 8 9 10 11 12 13 14 15 16 to 20

21 to 25 26 to 30 31 to 50 More than 50 men

PLEASE CHECK – Have you included ALL these men in Q.12, up to a maximum of 10?

16. Have you ever had treatment for a venereal disease (V.D.)?

Yes ☐   No ☐

If yes, have you ever had gonorrhoea?

Yes ☐   No ☐   Don't Know ☐

If you have had gonorrhoea: how many times have you had it? ☐

How old were you when you first had it? ☐

17. Have you ever had an abortion (i.e. induced pregnancy termination)?

Yes ☐   No ☐

18. Have you ever had anal intercourse with any of your **male** partners? (i.e. partner putting penis into back passage)

Yes ☐   No ☐

If yes, with how many of your male partners did you do this: ☐

Did you do this: Once only ☐   Occasionally ☐   Regularly ☐

THANK YOU FOR HELPING US.

Please ask the Interviewer if you did not understand how to fill in the answers or if you did not understand what any of the questions meant.

PLEASE SEAL YOUR QUESTIONNAIRE IN THE ENVELOPE AND PUT IT IN THE BOX.

THIS QUESTIONNAIRE IS CONFIDENTIAL AND ANONYMOUS – DO NOT GIVE YOUR NAME

Questionnaire for Men

1. What is your year of birth? . . . .

2. What is your job? . . . .

3. How old were you when you left school/fulltime education?

4. Did you get any qualifications and if so what? . . . .
    . . . .

5. What is your present marital status? *(Tick one)*

Single		Divorced		Widowed	
Married		Separated			

6. Who do you live with? *(Tick more than one if necessary)*

Alone		Wife		Friend(s)	
Parent(s)		Partner		Other	

7. Would you please answer some questions about any **marriages**, and **partners you have lived with**?

	What year did you start living with your wife or partner?	How lond did you live with your wife or partner?	Did you marry?
Wife or Partner 1			
,, ,, ,, 2			
,, ,, ,, 3			
,, ,, ,, 4			
,, ,, ,, 5			
,, ,, ,, 6			

8. How many children have you?

47

9. What is your ethnic group?

    European/White ☐   Indian/Pakistani/Bangladeshi ☐

    African/Afro-Caribbean ☐   Other ☐

First we would like to ask you about your sexual experiences with women

10. Have you ever had sexual intercourse with a woman?

    Yes ☐   No ☐

    If the answer is 'NO' go straight to question 17

11. How old were you when you first had intercourse? ☐

12. These questions are about the **last ten women** you have had sexual intercourse with.

    Include one night stands, casual and longer-term partners

    For each woman please fill in all of the boxes. Start with the woman you have most recently had sexual intercourse with.

	What year did you first have sexual intercourse with her?	Do you still have intercourse with her? *YES/NO*	If *NO*, how long did this sexual relationship last?	About how old was the woman at the start?	About how often do/did you have intercourse each month on average?	Do/did you use condoms *(ALWAYS, USUALLY, SOMETIMES, NEVER)*
Most recent						
One before						
One before						
One before						
One before						
One before						
One before						
One before						
One before						
One before						

The questions which follow on the next pages may seem similar and for some people the answers may be almost the same. They are however slightly different, in ways which can be important. Would you therefore please try to **answer them all** *as carefully as you can?*

13. *How many* **new** *sexual partners have you had in each of the* **last six years**?

Include one night stands, casual and longer-term partners

Year

1991	☐
1990	☐
1989	☐
1988	☐
1987	☐
1986	☐

Place a Number or (0)
in each box

14. People often have different numbers of sexual relationships during different ages in their life. We need to find out about this.

How many **new** sexual partners did you have when you were aged:–

Include one night stands, casual and longer-term partners

17 yrs or less	☐
18-19 years	☐
20-24 years	☐
25-29 years	☐
30-34 years	☐
35-39 years	☐
40-44 years	☐
45-49 years	☐
50 yrs or more	☐

*Place a Number or (0)
in each box up to your
present age*

15. About how many women have you had intercourse with **in your life**?
    (Please ring whichever number is applicable)

    1 2 3 4 5 6 7 8 9 10 11 12 13 14 15 16 to 20

    21 to 25   26 to 30   31 to 50   More than 50 women

PLEASE CHECK – Have you included ALL these women in Q.12, up to a maximum of 10?

16. Have you ever had sexual intercourse with a prostitute?

    Yes ☐   No ☐

    If yes, how many times did this occur when you were aged:–

17 yrs or less	☐
18-19 years	☐
20-24 years	☐
25-29 years	☐
30-34 years	☐
35-39 years	☐
40-44 years	☐
45-49 years	☐
50 yrs or more	☐

    Place a Number or (0) in each box up to your present age

Now we would like to ask you about your sexual experiences with men
Please answer **every** question

17. Have you ever had any kind of sexual experience with another man?

    Yes ☐   No ☐

18. Have you ever had anal intercourse with another man?

    Yes ☐   No ☐

19. How old were you the first time you had anal intercourse with another man?

Age [   ]   Never [   ]

20. How old were you the last time you had anal intercourse with another man?

Age [   ]   Never [   ]

21. About how many men have you had anal intercourse with **in your life**?
(Please ring whichever number is applicable)

1   2   3   4   5   6   7   8   9   10   11   12   13   14   15   16 to 20

21 to 25   26 to 30   31 to 50   More than 50 men

22. If you have ever had anal intercourse with another man were you?

always the passive partner   [   ]

usually the passive partner   [   ]

equally passive and active   [   ]

usually the active partner   [   ]

always the active partner   [   ]

never had anal intercourse with a man [   ]

23. Have you ever had anal intercourse with a male prostitute?

Yes [   ]   No [   ]

Finally we would like everyone to answer the following questions

24. Have you ever had treatment for a venereal disease (V.D.)?

Yes [   ]   No [   ]

If Yes, have you ever had gonorrhea?

Yes [   ]   No [   ]   Don't know [   ]

If you have had gonorrhoea:

How many times have you had it

How old were you when you first had it

25. Have you ever had anal intercourse with any of your **female** partners? (i.e. putting penis into partner's back passage)

Yes ☐   No ☐

If yes, with how many of your female partners did you do this: ☐

Did you do this: Once only ☐   Occasionally ☐   Regularly ☐

THANK YOU FOR HELPING US.

Please ask the Interviewer if you did not understand how to fill in the answers or if you did not understand what any of the questions meant.

PLEASE SEAL YOUR QUESTIONNAIRE IN THE ENVELOPE AND PUT IT IN THE BOX.

Chapter 8 – The Sample and its Characteristics

Assembling a Sample

We knew from the beginning that there was no way of obtaining a perfect sample. Access would not be allowed to local Family Practitioner Committee Registers (10) or the Central NHS Register at Southport. Electoral registers are always partly out of date, especially in the important early age groups, and they do not record ages. A postal enquiry based upon the Electoral Register or upon the Central Postcode Directory, and directed impersonally to those over 18 (say), would probably yield such a poor response rate that door-to-door enquiries would be needed. We were uncertain about response rates, even here, not to mention difficulties of access when potential respondents were out. The presence in the house of family members and doubts about anonymity would limit the degree of cooperation; and the costs would anyway be far beyond foreseeable resources.

We therefore decided upon a 'place of work' survey in which the sample would be assembled from a broad range of industrial, service-industry, commercial and educational environments, and would cover both private sector and public sector enterprises. The disadvantages were i) that such samples can be related to the general population only through indirect means: and ii) that the unemployed are specifically excluded – including housewives and retired persons and those engaged only in 'unofficial' occupations.

It was possible to 'patch' some of these deficiencies through samples taken from Institutes of Education: and to include unemployed young people registered for Youth Training Schemes (YTS) and housewives and retired individuals attending various courses. It was also possible to collect sufficient demographic and social data to relate our sample to the total population. None of these procedures completely repairs the defects, but the method offers two great advantages, probably sufficient to override its problems. The first is the evident anonymity of the process: in contrast with an interviewer or postal questionnaire arriving at the respondent's house. A visit depending on a known address does not visibly guarantee anonymity. The second is the absence of spouses, partners or other family members, the workplace providing social privacy in this respect. There were other benefits to this method. When the group negotiations were successful, the prevailing group ethic often yielded very high returns, circumventing the problem of having to rely upon 'volunteers', and avoiding the statistical hazards of an uncontrolled selective response. Finally, the approach promised economy in terms of completed histories per unit of resource – although this was in practice less clear-cut than we had anticipated.

Many different approaches and professional contacts were used to obtain introductions to factories, hospitals, technical colleges etc. This included searches facilitated by colleagues, but was generally based on a systematic approach to institutions listed in available registers. We would normally write a letter first and follow it up with an explanation of the study, by telephone. In favourable cases we would obtain an interview and explain our purposes to the managing director, the chief personnel officer, or other senior officer and/or the works doctor. At this stage they were shown the questionnaire forms and the rationale and practical details were explained. The forms were not shown in advance to potential respondents. The management staff would themselves usually undertake to negotiate with the work force, the union representatives and the shop stewards, to provide premises and to suggest suitable times. Once these agreements had been reached, the work force would attend in groups of ten to thirty, complete their forms, and return to work. Management staff often attended as well. The personnel director would supply the number of persons on the premises and therefore eligible to attend, so that we could compare this with the number who actually came. From this we could calculate the response rate.

Once people had attended and listened to the introductory talk, it was rare for them not to complete the questionnaire, fully and conscientiously. To encourage people to attend, they were informed in advance that initial attendance did not indicate commitment and that after listening to the talk, they would be given plenty of opportunity to opt out of completing a questionnaire. It was suggested that should they decide not to participate, the most private and easiest way of opting-out was to seal the blank questionnaire in the envelope, and wait until the end of the session to post it in the box along with everyone else. The portable screens meant that no one could observe whether a particular individual had or had not completed the questionnaire.

The overall recruitment process did not always work so smoothly. Although we had originally intended to recruit our respondents from institutions ranging from the very small to the very large, it emerged that for those employing less than around 100 people, there was a potential difficulty in providing objective and visible anonymity. It would sometimes have been technically possible to identify individuals from unique combinations of such items as age, gender, marital status, and ethnic group. It was made clear that identification would never be attempted, and that the data would never be seen by the management, but it must have been evident to those who thought about it that it *could* be done.

The very large firms were also unrewarding, for a different reason. Local factories and branches (e.g. of a department store or an insurance company) sometimes asked us to go through head office. More frequently than for local negotiations, this led to refusals, partly because the work patterns in such firms tend to be highly structured and therefore difficult to interrupt. Even where consent in principle was obtained, it was still necessary to undertake local negotiations as well, perhaps with several divisions, each with its own managers. These negotiations frequently grounded on cross purposes between different management levels. The success rate was low, and even where it was successful the negotiations often took many months, and neutralised the advantages of economy which the approach had seemed to offer.

Our most successful approaches (although not exclusively so) were to medium-sized firms and institutions or to specific sections within larger organisations. Once contact had been made with the work force or with their immediate representatives there were hardly any problems at all. There were no objections or obstructions, anywhere, from union representatives or shop stewards. With rare exceptions, the respondents completed their questionnaires in a responsible, serious, and non-jocular manner. Very few refused to attend and most of the non-responding fraction were missed through administrative hiccups or occasionally because a manager misunderstood or disregarded our careful explanations and asked for 'volunteers'.

The sample recruitment process suffered an interruption when there was political interference at the highest level with a national survey conducted from another centre. This was reported widely by the media and our investigation was misidentified with it. We also found other problems; some sources agreed to take part, but not in the holiday period (June-Sept) or in the busy months running up to Christmas (Oct-Dec) or at times approaching municipal elections. These types of delays were all temporary, but together they cost us some months and we found ourselves in an era where the enthusiasm for supporting research on this disease had declined, and where there was even some antipathy. We kept on trying, but with less success. Our last approach was a presentation to a convention of Personnel Managers from over 30 suitable firms. It was conducted under sympathetic chairmanship and was well received, but when the message was returned to the firms themselves there were no positive responses at all. At this stage, still short on numbers compared with our aspirations, we decided to stop.

Characteristics of the Sample

The main disadvantage of the institutional method of sampling was that the relationship between the sample and the population as a whole was not formally definable. However, the problem was ameliorated by measuring the differences between the sample and the general population in respect of those social and demographic characteristics for which national statistics were available. The social and demographic features of the sample are described below, together with an account of the selection biases of the sample-taking process.

The sample consisted of 2530 persons, 1289 males and 1241 females. They were contacted through a number of institutions with representatives in each of the following employment sectors: i) manufacturing industry, ii) service industry (e.g. insurance, retailing), iii)local or central government, iv) health services and v) those in full-time education. We also contacted persons in part-time education, often on release from employments in these other sectors. We also managed to include a number of unemployed and retired persons, and some housewives. Table 8.1 shows the numbers of men and women within each of these sectors.

Table 8.1

Numbers of Males and Females from each Employment Sector Source

Employment Sector	Males		Females		Total	
	n	%	n	%	n	%
Manufacturing industry	545	42.3	217	17.5	762	30.1
Service industry	170	13.2	255	20.5	425	16.8
Central & local government	180	14.0	257	20.7	437	17.3
Health services	56	4.3	178	14.3	234	9.2
Students	225	17.5	238	19.2	463	18.3
Unemployed/Retired	72	5.5	44	3.4	116	4.6
Housewife	–		22	1.8	22	0.9
Not known	41	3.2	30	2.4	71	2.8
Total	1289	100	1241	100	2530	100

The manufacturing sector supplied the largest proportion (42.3%) of the men while the different service industry sources, including Central/local government and health service sectors, supplied the largest proportion of the women (55.5%). The educational sector supplied similar proportions of full-time male and female students. The 'unemployed' category included 15 men who were retired. None of the women classified themselves as 'retired', but rather as unemployed or housewives.

Table 8.2 shows the numbers of men and women from each source within different age bands. Among the men, those contacted through service industries, central/local government and health services tended to be older, while those in manufacturing industry, and more especially the students, were concentrated in the lower age bands. Among the females the different sources were more evenly distributed, apart from the students.

Table 8.2

Employment sector sources and age of respondents

Males
Age Group (yrs)

Source	Under 19	19-20	21-22	23-24	25-30	31-45	46+	N/K	Total
Manufacturing industry	188	68	39	28	46	99	75	2	545
Service industry	15	25	20	11	36	43	20	–	170
Central & local government	6	11	14	15	42	67	24	1	180
Health services	6	14	8	2	5	14	6	1	56
Students	123	66	12	7	8	4	–	5	225
Unemployed/Retired	19	8	7	1	14	11	11	1	72
Not known	16	1	5	4	1	6	–	8	41
Total	373	193	105	68	152	244	136	18	1289
(%)	(28.9)	(15.1)	(8.1)	(5.3)	(11.8)	(18.9)	(10.6)	(1.4)	(100)

Females
Age Group (yrs)

Source	Under 19	19-20	21-22	23-24	25-30	31-45	46+	N/K	Total
Manufacturing industry	37	28	26	17	38	42	28	1	217
Service industry	26	41	34	30	51	60	11	2	255
Central & local government	3	12	22	27	75	77	38	3	257
Health services	9	23	18	13	28	70	17	–	178
Students	105	63	23	11	19	14	2	1	238
Unemployed	8	9	5	2	13	3	3	–	44
Housewives	–	–	1	–	5	16	–	–	22
Not known	7	3	5	4	5	4	2	–	30
Total	195	179	134	105	234	286	101	7	1241
(%)	(15.7)	(14.4)	(10.8)	(8.5)	(18.9)	(23.0)	(8.1)	(0.6)	(100)

The majority of respondents (69%) were aged 30 or less, differing in this respect from the adult population as a whole. However, provided that proper allowance was made, this was to the benefit of the investigation because it turned out that these were the ages in which the most relevant sexual activities were concentrated. Indeed, when the early results had indicated how important the younger age groups were, recruitment from sources where these groups were widely available was deliberately expanded.

Table 8.3 distributes respondents from different sectors according to the Registrar-General's Classification of occupations. Among the men, the manufacturing sector

Table 8.3

Employment Sector Sources According to Social Class

Males
Social Class

Source	I, II	IIINM	IIIM	IV, V	Unclassified	Total
Manufacturing industry	79	62	362	27	15	545
Service industry	69	62	11	19	9	170
Central & local government	68	102	1	2	7	180
Health services	25	2	25	3	1	56
Students	1	–	1	–	223	225
Unemployed/Retired	2	3	3	1	63	72
Not Known	–	1	–	–	40	41
Total	244	232	403	52	358	1289
(%)	(18.9)	(18.0)	(31.3)	(4.0)	(27.8)	(100)

Females*
Social Class

Source	I, II	IIINM	IIIM	IV, V	Unclassified	Total
Manufacturing industry	73	67	40	23	14	217
Service industry	48	175	13	13	6	255
Central & local government	75	165	7	5	5	257
Health services	124	24	18	8	4	178
Students	–	–	–	–	238	238
Unemployed	–	–	–	–	42	44
Housewives	1	1	–	–	21	22
Not Known	–	–	–	–	30	30
Total	321	432	78	49	361	1241
(%)	(25.9)	(34.8)	(6.3)	(3.2)	(29.1)	(100)

*Based on woman's own occupation

Table 8.4

Employment Sector Source and Age at completing full-time education

Males
Age at completing FTE

Source	16 or less	17-19	20+	Still** there	N/K	Total
Manufacturing industry	424	101	12	3	5	545
Service industry	69	69	29	2	1	170
Central/local government	72	57	47	1	3	180
Health services	24	26	6	–	–	56
Students*	61	15	–	145	4	225
Unemployed/Retired	45	16	7	2	2	72
Not Known	21	9	–	1	10	41
Total	716	293	101	154	25	1289
(%)	(55.5)	(22.7)	(7.8)	(11.9)	(1.9)	(100)

Females
Age at completing FTE

Source	16 or less	17-19	20+	Still** there	N/K	Total
Manufacturing industry	142	69	3	–	2	217
Service industry	127	108	15	1	3	255
Central/local government	116	87	50	–	1	257
Health services	81	82	13	2	–	178
Students*	49	27	2	138	22	238
Unemployed	19	18	3	2	2	44
Housewives	13	8	1	–	–	22
Not known	16	6	1	–	7	30
Total	563	405	88	143	37	1241
(%)	(45.4)	(32.6)	(7.1)	(11.5)	(3.0)	(100)

*Some full-time students had left school and returned to full-time education later. Some had obviously misunderstood the question and answered for the age at which they left school.

**A few were in F.T.E. seconded by employer

Table 8.5

Social Class & Age at Completing Full-time Education

Males
Age at completing FTE

Social Class	16 or less	17-19	20+	Still there**	N/K	Total
I & II	82	96	65	–	1	244
IIINM	130	81	18	1	2	232
IIIM	335	59	6	1	2	403
IV & V	34	16	1	–	1	52
Unclassified	135	41	10	152	20	358
Total	716	293	98	154	26	1289
(%)	(55.5)	(22.7)	(7.6)	(11.9)	(2.0)	(100)

Females
Age at completing FTE

Social Class*	16 or less	17-19	20+	Still there**	N/K	Total
I & II	107	146	67	1	–	321
IIINM	243	167	19	–	3	432
IIIM	58	18	1	–	1	78
IV & V	44	5	–	–	–	49
Unclassified	111	69	6	143	32	361
Total	563	405	88	144	36	1241
(%)	(45.4)	(32.6)	(7.1)	(11.6)	(2.9)	(100)

*Based on woman's own occupation

**A few were in F.T.E. seconded by employer

supplied relatively few respondents from Social Classes I and II: while the different service sectors were more heavily represented in this respect. The women did not show the same contrast between manufacturing industry on the one hand, and the service industries and Central and Local Government on the other. However, female respondents contacted through the health service sources showed a very high proportion from Social Classes I and II. The social class for females that is referred to throughout the monograph was based on their own occupations.

The relationships between the different employment sources and ages at completion of full-time education are shown in Table 8.4, for men and for women separately. The greatest proportions of early school leavers were from the manufacturing industries, and later completion of full-time education at age 20 or older was especially associated with the central/local government sector. The patterns here were similar for men and for women, although the differences were a little more marked for the men.

The different social indices were themselves inter-related as illustrated in Tables 8.5 and 8.6. Table 8.5 shows the relationship between social class and the age at completion of full-time education. Table 8.6 shows the relationship between social

Table 8.6

Social Class and Educational Qualifications

Males

Social Class	None	Voc/CSE/ 'O'-level**	'A'** level	Higher	N/K	Total
I,II	19	79	36	105	5	244
IIINM	24	141	36	23	8	232
IIIM	98	259	8	10	28	403
IV,V	22	18	6	4	2	52
Unclassified	35	208	55	16	44	358
Total	198	705	141	158	87	1289
(%)	(15.4)	(54.7)	(10.9)	(12.3)	(6.7)	(100)

Females

Social Class*	None	Voc/CSE/ 'O'-level**	'A'** level	Higher	N/K	Total
I,II	17	151	55	94	4	321
IIINM	46	282	56	29	19	432
IIIM	22	43	3	2	8	78
IV,V	27	15	2	–	5	49
Unclassified	29	182	79	18	53	361
Total	141	673	195	143	89	1241
(%)	(11.4)	(54.2)	(15.7)	(11.5)	(7.2)	(100)

*Based on woman's own occupation

**Some qualifications were equivalent to these

class and the highest level of educational qualifications obtained. As might be expected, Social Classes I and II had completed their fulltime education relatively late; and greater proportions of Social Classes I, II and III-non-manual had attained 'A'-level qualifications or higher.

Respondents were asked to declare their ethnic group, and 98.3% of the men and 99.5% of the women gave this information. The few blank entries were probably intended – at our own suggestion – as a device for protecting anonymity. Among those who gave ethnic group information, 74.2 percent of the males and 67.9 percent of the females classified themselves as European/White. Most of the remainder said they were African/Afro-Caribbean or Indian/Pakistani/Bangladeshi. The Afro-Caribbeans constituted only 5.5 percent of the males but 15.3 percent of the females. Indo/Pakistanis constituted 15.8 percent of the males and 12.7 percent of the females. Social class distributions by ethnic group in males and in females are shown in Table 8.7.

Table 8.7

Social Class and Ethnic Group

Males

Social Class	Cauc	Afro/Car	Indo/Pak	Other	N/K	Total
I,II	221	10	11	2	–	244
IIINM	199	17	9	2	5	232
IIIM	359	14	19	5	6	403
IV,V	36	5	9	2	–	52
Unclassified	141	25	156	25	11	358
Total	956	71	204	36	22	1289
(%)	(74.2)	(5.5)	(15.8)	(2.8)	(1.7)	(100.0)

Females

Social Class*	Cauc	Afro/Car	Indo/Pak	Other	N/K	Total
I,II	272	25	19	5	–	321
IIINM	328	64	31	8	1	432
IIIM	61	8	5	3	1	78
IV,V	42	4	3	–	–	49
Unclassified	140	89	99	29	4	361
Total	843	190	157	45	6	1241
(%)	(67.9)	(15.3)	(12.7)	(3.6)	(0.5)	(100.0)

*Based on woman's own occupation

Table 8.8

Age of Respondents and Ethnic Group

Age Group	Males					
(yrs)	Cauc	Afro/Car	Indo/Pak	Other	N/K	Total
Under 19	253	9	91	14	6	373
19,20	112	15	59	6	1	193
21,22	76	10	14	2	3	105
23,24	50	7	5	6	–	68
25-30	121	13	11	3	4	152
31-45	222	10	10	1	1	244
46+	117	4	12	1	2	136
N/K	5	3	2	3	5	18
Total	956	71	204	36	22	1289
(%)	(74.2)	(5.5)	(15.8)	(2.8)	(1.7)	(100.0)

Age Group	Females					
(yrs)	Cauc	Afro/Car	Indo/Pak	Other	N/K	Total
Under 19	91	24	64	16	–	195
19,20	100	25	42	12	–	179
21,22	73	29	27	3	2	134
23,24	77	18	9	1	–	105
25-30	162	57	7	8	–	234
31-45	237	34	8	4	3	286
46+	98	2	–	–	1	101
N/K	5	1	–	1	–	7
Total	843	190	157	45	6	1241
(%)	(67.9)	(15.3)	(12.7)	(3.6)	(0.5)	(100.0)

There was a relative deficiency of Social Classes I and II among non-Caucasian males, particularly among the Indo/Pakistanis; the pattern was similar among the females. The Indo/Pakistani respondents, both males and females, tended to be younger than the Caucasians and Afro-Caribbeans (Table 8.8). Table 8.9 shows the educational qualifications attained in the different ethnic groups. The general levels were similar,

Table 8.9

Educational Qualification and Ethnic Group

Qualification Group	Males					
	Cauc	Afro/Car	Indo/Pak	Other	N/K	Total
None	156	14	21	2	5	198
Voc/CSE/O level*	509	41	122	24	9	705
A level*	104	7	23	6	1	141
Higher	141	4	11	2	–	158
N/K	46	5	27	2	7	87
Total	956	71	204	36	22	1289
(%)	(74.2)	(5.5)	(15.8)	(2.8)	(1.7)	(100)

Qualification Group	Females					
	Cauc	Afro/Car	Indo/Pak	Other	N/K	Total
None	110	18	8	5	–	141
Voc/CSE/O level*	431	129	83	28	2	673
A level*	142	19	27	7	–	195
Higher	121	9	13	–	–	143
N/K	39	15	26	5	4	89
Total	843	190	157	45	6	1241
(%)	(67.9)	(15.3)	(12.7)	(3.6)	(0.5)	(100)

*Some qualifications were equivalent to these

although the Caucasians had greater numbers reporting the highest qualifications, both in males and females.

The other main recorded demographic variables were marital status and number of children. The distribution according to marital status is shown in Table 8.10; and according to the number of children, in Table 8.11. Most respondents (68.3 percent of the men and 65.4 percent of the women) were single. The majority (72.5 percent of the men and 69.5 percent of the women) had no children. These figures reflect the early age distribution of our sample.

Table 8.10

Marital Status

Marital Status	Males		Females		Total	
	number	percent	number	percent	number	percent
Single	880	68.3	811	65.4	1691	66.8
Married	364	28.2	330	26.6	694	27.4
Divorced	21	1.6	61	4.9	82	3.2
Separated	16	1.2	23	1.9	39	1.5
Widowed	4	0.3	11	0.9	15	0.6
N/K	4	0.3	5	0.4	9	0.3

Table 8.11

Number of Children

No. children	Males		Females		Total	
	number	percent	number	percent	number	percent
0	935	72.5	862	69.5	1797	71.0
1	91	7.1	123	9.9	214	8.5
2	172	13.3	178	14.3	350	13.9
3	56	4.3	51	4.1	107	4.2
4	17	1.3	21	1.7	38	1.5
5	7	0.5	3	0.2	10	0.4
6+	5	0.4	2	0.2	7	0.3
N/K	6	0.5	1	0.1	7	0.3

Table 8.12

Social Class and Marital Status

	Males				
Social Class	Single	Married	Div/Sep/Wid	N/K	Total
I,II	112	123	9	–	244
IIINM	149	74	9	–	232
IIIM	282	111	8	2	403
IV,V	29	18	5	–	52
Unclassified	308	88	10	2	358
Total	880	364	41	4	1289
(%)	(68.3)	(28.2)	(3.2)	(0.3)	(100)

Table 8.12 cont.

Social Class*	Single	Married	Div/Sep/Wid	N/K	Total
			Females		
I,II	183	106	32	–	321
IIINM	261	129	40	2	432
IIIM	49	22	6	1	78
IV,V	18	26	5	–	49
Unclassified	300	47	12	2	361
Total	811	330	95	5	1241
(%)	(65.4)	(26.6)	(7.7)	(0.4)	(100)

*Based on woman's own occupation

Table 8.13

Social Class and Children

Social Class	No Children	Children	N/K	Total
		Males		
I, II	150	94	–	244
IIINM	160	72	–	232
IIIM	290	113	–	403
IV, V	27	25	–	52
Unclassified	308	44	6	358
Total	935	348	6	1289
(%)	(72.5)	(27.0)	(0.5)	(100)

Social Class*	No Children	Children	N/K	Total
		Females		
I, II	215	106	–	321
IIINM	301	131	–	432
IIIM	40	30	–	78
IV, V	16	33	–	49
Unclassified	282	78	1	361
Total	862	378	1	1241
(%)	(69.5)	(30.5)	(0.1)	(100)

*Based on woman's own occupation

Table 8.12 and Table 8.13 show the ways in which marital status and numbers of children related to Social Class. Men in Social Classes I and II were more often married than single: with the reverse in the other classes and in the unclassified. Relatively few women in Social Classes IV, V and unclassified were married. The unclassified group was dominated by full-time students most of whom were single. The proportion of respondents with children varied little according to social class, except for a very low rate among the unclassified group. Table 8.14 shows the association between age and marital status. Almost all respondents up to the age of 24 were single; while from 31 years onwards the majority were or had been married.

Table 8.14

Age of Respondent and Marital Status

Males

Age group (yrs)	Single	Married	Div/Sep/Wid	N/K	Total
Under 19	369	1	1	2	373
19-20	187	3	3	–	193
21-22	100	4	1	–	105
23-24	58	10	–	–	68
25-30	94	50	8	–	152
31-45	53	174	17	–	244
46+	6	120	10	–	136
N/K	13	2	1	2	18
Total	880	364	41	4	1289
(%)	(68.3)	(28.2)	(3.2)	(0.3)	(100)

Females

Age group (yrs)	Single	Married	Div/Sep/Wid	N/K	Total
Under 19	193	2	–	–	54
19-20	173	4	2	–	179
21-22	119	13	1	1	134
23-24	91	10	4	–	105
25-30	140	84	9	1	234
31-45	78	150	51	3	286
46+	14	64	16	–	101
N/K	3	3	1	–	7
Total	811	330	84	11	1241
(%)	(65.4)	(26.6)	(6.8)	(0.4)	(100)

The relationships between ethnic group and marital status is shown in Table 8.15 and between ethnic group and number of children in Table 8.16. Far more of the married and the divorced/separated/widowed respondents were Caucasian. More Caucasian as well as Afro-Caribbean respondents had children when compared with the Indo/Pakistani respondents; and this was so both for men and for women.

National Comparisons

The sample is better described as 'broad ranging' than truly representative of the general population. However, the number of individual sources and the spread of occupational classes were sufficient to limit the effects of any idiosyncratic bias in

Table 8.15

Ethnic Group and Marital Status

Males

Ethnic Group	Single	Married	Div/Sep/Wid	N/K	Total
Caucasian	599	321	34	2	956
Afro/Car	57	8	6	–	71
Ind/Pak	176	28	–	–	204
Other	31	4	1	–	36
N/K	17	3	–	2	22
Total	880	364	41	4	1289
(%)	(68.3)	(28.2)	(3.2)	(0.3)	(100)

Females

Ethnic Group	Single	Married	Div/Sep/Wid	N/K	Total
Caucasian	469	284	87	3	843
Afro/Car	166	21	2	1	190
Ind/Pak	134	22	5	–	147
Other	39	4	1	1	45
N/K	3	3	–	–	6
Total	811	330	95	5	1241
(%)	(65.4)	(26.6)	(7.7)	(0.4)	(100)

Table 8.16

Ethnic Group and Children

Ethnic Group	Males			
	No Children	**Children**	**N/K**	**Total**
Caucasian	660	295	1	956
Afro/Car	53	17	1	71
Ind/Pak	175	27	2	204
Other	32	4	–	36
N/K	15	5	2	22
Total	935	348	6	1289
(%)	(72.5)	(27.0)	(0.5)	(100)

Ethnic Group	Females			
	No Children	**Children**	**N/K**	**Total**
Caucasian	557	286	–	843
Afro/Car	123	67	–	190
Ind/Pak	141	16	–	157
Other	38	7	–	45
N/K	3	2	1	6
Total	862	378	1	1241
(%)	(69.5)	(30.5)	(0.1)	(100)

different parts of the sample. The total group might therefore be regarded as a reasonably representative sample – at least of the working population – although the manner of our approach would almost certainly have involved differential sampling ratios in the different sub-strata. Our next task is to characterise the nature, the degree and the effects of this stratification through comparing our own results with those observed in the population at large.

The proportional ethnic mix for the United Kingdom is officially reported (11) in 1987-89 as constituting 1.11 percent West Indian, Guyanese or African: 2.42 percent Indian, Pakistani or Bangladeshi: and 1.17 percent other ethnic minority groups. These proportions are larger in the West Midlands, as is reflected in our sample (percentages in Table 8.7). For extrapolating results to the country as a whole, although not necessarily to other large cities, it would therefore be necessary to down-grade weightings attached to the findings in non-Caucasian groups.

The Social Class distribution of the sample can be compared with the UK distribution of the socio-economic groups of a sample of heads of households in the period 1989-90 (11: Table 2.6). This national sample showed 25.6 percent in Social Classes I and II together, 20.9 percent and 30.5 percent in Classes IIINM and IIIM and 16.9 percent and 5.7 percent in the semi-skilled and unskilled manual classes IV and V. Excluding the unemployed, the students, and those who did not record their occupation, the corresponding distribution for men in our own sample was 26.2 (I + II), 24.9 (IIINM), 43.3 (IIIM), 4.5 (IV) and 1.1 (V) percent. This shows a relative deficiency among Social Classes IV and V. Among the women, the sample was less appropriately compared with a 'Head of Household' distribution; and, in addition, the women in the sample were categorised according to their own occupations and not that of their husband's or partner's. The respective percentages were 36.5, 49.1, 8.9, 5.2 and 0.3 percent, again indicating low proportions in the less affluent groups. Extrapolations from the sample of any sexual behaviour findings which show a social gradient, will require increased weighting of the levels and styles of these less affluent classes.

The largest proportion of the men in our sample, 42.3 percent, were engaged in manufacturing industry. For the females, 17.5 percent were so engaged. For both sexes together the overall proportion was 30.1%. In the United Kingdom as a whole, 5.15 millions out of 22.86 millions in employment (22.5 percent) were employed thus. (11: Table 4.1). The excess in our study may be related partly to our recruitment methods, but it also reflects the fact that the investigation was conducted in an industrial area. This too must be taken into account in any attempted extrapolations.

In 1988-1990 in Great Britain (11: Table 3.3), 14 percent of the white population had obtained a higher educational qualification: 32 percent achieved no educational qualifications: and the remaining 55 percent attained an intermediate level. Attainments were slightly better for males than for females. Among Afro-Caribbeans, nationally, 11 percent had achieved a higher qualification, 34 percent none, and 55 percent an intermediate level. Among Indians, 16 percent had achieved a higher qualification, 36 percent none, and 49 percent an intermediate level. Among Pakistani/Bangladeshi immigrants the situation was worse with only 6 percent attaining a higher qualification; while 60 percent achieved none. 'Other' minority ethnic groups did best of all: 21 percent achieved a higher qualification and only 25 percent did not achieve any.

The respondents in our sample had done better than the national population. In particular, smaller proportions achieved no educational qualifications: only 15.4 percent of the men and 11.4 percent of the women *(see Table 8.6)*. The lowest proportion of 'nil' qualifications was in the Indo-Pakistani ethnic group. *(see Table 8.9)*. This contrasts with the national figures. These favourable levels of performance are presumably a function of the fact that our sample consisted of people in work: and

Table 8.17

Response levels and sexual behaviour

Males (initiated with either sex)	High response	Medium response	Low response
No. of cases*	799	201	82
1st heterosexual intercourse <18 years (%)**	66.3	38.9	51.2
Total heterosexual partners (mean)**	6.0	6.2	8.1
Heterosexual anal sex (%)**	22.4	11.8	15.6
Use of prostitute (%)**	6.7	10.1	13.4
Homosexual relationship (%)	7.3	8.2	3.8
Homosexual anal sex (%)	3.7	4.6	1.3
Sexually transmitted disease (%)	6.2	4.1	6.3

*16 cases initiated with a male only

**includes only those males initiated with a female

Females (initiated)	High response	Medium response	Low response
No. of cases	792	122	82
1st heterosexual intercourse <18 years (%)	51.8	29.5	60.5
Total heterosexual partners (mean)	3.9	3.2	4.7
Heterosexual anal sex (%)	17.1	15.8	25.0
Pregnancy termination (%)	18.4	15.8	13.6
Sexually transmitted disease (%)	6.2	1.6	2.4

perhaps also of the type of work associated with successful recruitment. The younger age distribution of our sample, and the use of educational institutes for recruitment, would also contribute to the lower proportions with no educational qualifications.

Responder Self-selection

The need to avoid responder self-selection had greatly influenced the design of the study. It was one of the main reasons for adopting work-place sampling. If response rates within institutions were great enough, there would be little scope for behaviour-related bias. The data were examined to see whether there were any systematic variations of sexual history associated with these different levels of response.

We calculated response rates for each institution, ascertaining the number of individuals available to take part, and comparing it with the number who completed a questionnaire. The responses for the different institutions were then classified into 'high', 'medium' or 'low'. 'High' meant 75% or more of the available individuals had taken part, the actual values ranging from 75% up to 96%. 'Medium' response rates were defined as 30-74%, ranging in fact from 45% to 51%. A 'low' response was defined as below 30%, the actual values ranging from 25% down to one institution with only a 6% response rate.

The pooled sexual behaviour records of the different response-rate groups are given in Table 8.17. This showed that there were no systematic differences between the high, medium or low response groups in respect of their sexual behaviour characteristics. This applied to both males and females. High levels of social confounding obviously hamper any firm conclusions, but there was no evidence here that low responses had selectively excluded those with extreme patterns of sexual behaviour, ie those with either higher or lower risks. In any case most respondents had come from the high response institutions.

Conclusions

The sampling difficulties were severe. There was no way, within foreseeable resources and an appropriate timescale, of coping with all of them. A search for advantages in one respect would always have to be bought at the expense of disadvantages in another respect. The 'place of work' approach was adopted largely because it offered relief from the hazards of a self-selected panel of respondents, of inhibited or untruthful replies arising from fears about privacy or personal identification, or the embarrassing presence of family members. The main disadvantage was the sacrifice of a formally representative sampling rule and, in the event, the sample was biased in several demonstrable ways. The main biases were with respect to the age distribution (too young) and the marital/demographic distributions (too many single and too many without children). Compared with national data there were fewer in Social Classes IV and V and more in IIINM. The ethnic mix was reasonable for the West Midlands, but biased with respect to the country as a whole. As regards forms of employment, manufacturing industry was over-represented among the men, as one might expect in the West Midlands; and education levels and educational attendance were greater than for the country as a whole.

The sample under-represented the very small and the very large organisations, and (probably) a range of lower paid jobs in highly- structured labour-intensive industries. It was also deficient with respect to the unemployed and those in mobile and dispersed occupations; also housewives, and those engaged only in home-based or 'unofficial' activities.

However, many of these sampling biases are capable of partial correction through reference to national data, and through an examination of the ways in which these factors influence sexual behaviour patterns. This is the task of the next chapter.

Chapter 9 – Sexual Behaviour among Respondents

This chapter describes the overall pattern of sexual behaviour among those who completed the questionnaires. It sets out the questions asked and explains their rationale. It then enumerates the different forms of reply.

If we are to relate the behaviour of this group to that of the population at large, we shall have to correct for the social and demographic biases already described. To do this it will be necessary to measure the extent to which sexual behaviour itself varies in these same social and demographic terms. These variations are also described.

However, social and demographic correction-procedures are not in themselves sufficient. It would be possible to select a sample which was socially and demographically representative, and without significant response bias, yet which was sexually atypical. For example, there were no whole-time prostitutes among those accessed through 'indoor' places of work; nor were the current and previous sexual activities of married women living at home, and not engaged in paid work, well represented within our groups. Our sampling method did not reach those in mobile or dispersed occupations – long-distance transport drivers, taxi drivers, bus and train drivers, mariners, milkmen, postmen, meter-readers, delivery-men, miners, farm workers, shop assistants and sales representatives. We had attempted to include some of these groups but came up against many problems which prevented access. The highly structured nature of the work in many labour-intensive industries, for example sales assistants in department stores and chain-stores, made contact difficult and costly, and employers refused access. In the dispersed occupations it was impossible to gather together enough individuals to provide visible anonymity; while homeless people and the unemployed, especially young mobile unemployed people, the armed services, the chronically sick and disabled, drug addicts, and prison populations, were excluded or under-represented.

Some of the above groups are traditionally regarded as relatively promiscuous. In addition – and as we shall demonstrate – there were wide personal variations in this respect among the groups to which we did indeed have access. For these two reasons, we questioned our respondents regarding certain indicators of high risk sexual activity. The purpose was to amplify the behavioural characterisation of this population subset. We asked whether they had had a venereal disease: and specifically gonorrhoea. If they had had it, how many times had they had it? We also asked the women whether they had had a termination of pregnancy; and if so, on how many occasions. We also hoped that these data would enable us to check our sample against available population statistics although, in the event, this was possible only in very general terms, because we were unable to find national data displayed in exactly comparable formats.

The Questions Asked

We asked six 'simple' questions demanding either a yes/no answer, or a single number, or a choice of categories to be 'ringed'. We also asked five complex questions, requiring entry of material in a tabular format. In addition, we asked two further sets of questions of the male respondents regarding a) homosexual behaviour and b) use of female and male prostitutes; and there was a special question for female respondents regarding pregnancy terminations which they had undergone. The exact layout of these questions is shown in Appendix A7. The essential enquiries were as follows.

The Six Simple Questions Were:

Q5. What is your present marital status? (single/married/divorced/separated/widowed).

Q6. Who do you live with? (alone/parents/wife/partner/friend/other).

Q8. How many children do you have?

Q10. Have you ever had sexual intercourse with a woman? (. . . or with a man, in the case of a female respondent). (yes/no).

Q11. (If yes to Q10) How old were you when you first had intercourse?

Q15. About how many women(/men) have you had intercourse with in your life? Please ring whichever number is applicable.

The Five Complex Questions:

Q7. Would you please answer some questions about any marriages, and partners you have lived with?

> For each wife/husband or other live-in partner the respondent was asked to enter to a table
> a) the year in which he/she started living with the partner:
> b) the duration of the living arrangement:
> c) whether they married.
> Sufficient space was provided for up to 6 spouses or live-in partners.

Q12. These questions are about the last ten women you have had sexual intercourse with. (. . . or ten men, in the case of a female respondent). Include one night stands. For each woman (/man), please fill in all the boxes. Start with the woman(/man) you have most recently had sexual intercourse with.

For each partner the respondent was asked to:
a) state the calendar year in which he/she first had sexual intercourse:
b) whether he/she still had intercourse with her/him (yes/no):
c) if no, how long the relationship lasted:
d) how old was the partner at the start:
e) how often do/did they have intercourse each month, on average:
f) do/did they use condoms? (always/usually/sometimes/never).

Space was provided for up to ten partners beginning with the most recent and moving backwards in time.

The questionnaire then gave the following instruction*

. 'The questions which follow on the next pages may seem similar and for some people the answers may be almost the same. They are however slightly different, in ways which can be important. Would you therefore please try to answer them all as carefully as you can?

Q.13 How many *new* sexual partners have you had in each of the last six years? Include one night stands, casual and longer-term partners. Place a number (or 0) in each box.

Space was provided for 6 entries, the boxes being labelled with the last six calendar years.

Q14. People often have different numbers of sexual relationships at different ages in their life. We need to find out about this. Include one night stands, casual and longer-term partners. How many *new* sexual partners did you have when you were aged:-

Nine boxes were provided labelled 17 years or less, 18-19, 20-24, 25-29, 30-34, 35-39, 40-44, 45-49, 50 years or more. Respondents were asked to place a number (or 0) in each box up to their present age.

*Verbal instructions had already been given for these questions by the researcher as part of the introductory talk.

Special Questions

Male respondents were asked:

Q16. Have you ever had sexual intercourse with a prostitute? (yes/no).

If yes, how many times did this occur when you were aged:-

The format of the panel was the same as that for Q14.

Q17. Have you ever had any kind of sexual experience with another man?

Q18. Have you ever had anal intercourse with another man?

Q19. How old were you when this *first* occurred?

Q20. How old were you when this *last* occurred?

Q21. About how many men have you had anal intercourse with in your life? Please ring whichever number is applicable.

Q22. Were you always/usually/equally the passive partner?

Q23. Have you ever had anal intercourse with a male prostitute?

Female respondents were asked:

Q17. Have you ever had an abortion (pregnancy termination)?

Both males and females were asked:

Q24(M) Q 16(F) Have you ever had treatment for a veneral disease? (If Yes details were requested.)

Q25(M) Q 18(F) Have you ever had anal intercourse with any of your female/male (heterosexual) partners? (If Yes details were requested.)

The Broad Pattern of Sexual Activity

Most of the respondents in this sample had had sexual intercourse with a member of the opposite sex. 1066 of the 1279 men who answered the question (83.3 percent) claimed to have had sexual intercourse with a woman; and 996 of the 1233 women (80.8 percent) claimed to have had sexual intercourse with a man.

Age of First Intercourse

Ages at first heterosexual intercourse for men and for women are given in Table 9.1, and the form of the distribution is shown in Figure 9.1. Such statistics are of limited value without a simultaneous consideration of the numbers of persons at risk, – a point we develop later. However, the peak age appeared to be lower for the boys (age 16) than for the girls (age 17). As many as 26.2% of the non-celibate males claimed that they first had intercourse at under the age of 16, and 14% of the females.

Table 9.1

	Age at First Intercourse*	
Age	**Males**	**Females**
<10	5	2
10	3	1
11	5	0
12	9	2
13	33	11
14	79	35
15	145	88
16	206	170
17	155	186
18	130	179
19	78	104
20	58	80
21	38	47
22	26	28
23	23	15
24	21	9
25	13	7
26	7	15
27	10	6
28	7	3
29	5	1
30-34	6	2
>34	2	2
never	211	235
N/K	14	13
Total	1289	1241

*This question was directed to first heterosexual intercouse but some may have misunderstood. Includes some cases of child abuse. We did not ask but some volunteered the information.

Figure 9.1

Age at First Intercourse

Males and Females.

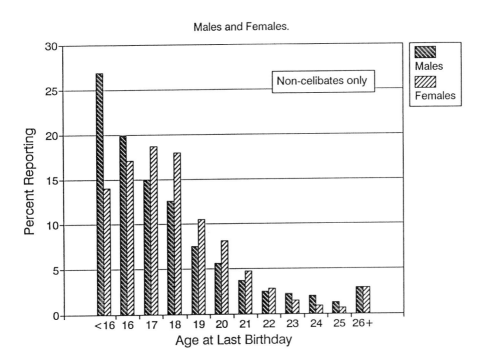

Total Lifetime Partners

Respondents were asked to state the number of heterosexual partners with whom they had had intercourse at any time during their lives. The full distribution is shown in Table 9.2 for men and for women separately. The overall mean value for men among those who had ever had a partner (sexually initiated) was 6.20 partners; and for women, 3.90 partners. These numbers refer to incomplete sexual careers, intercepted by the date of the enquiry, and the final numbers for completed sexual careers will inevitably be larger. The distribution was highly skewed. Among those who gave information on total number of partners 24.3 percent of the sexually initiated males and 31.1 percent of sexually initiated females had had only one partner at the time of the enquiry; but 6.1 percent of the initiated males and 2.0 percent of the females had had more than 20 lifetime partners.

Table 9.2

Total Heterosexual Partners

Number of Partners	Males		Females	
	n	%	n	%
0	215	17.1	236	19.4
1	253	20.1	306	25.1
2	149	11.9	222	18.2
3	132	10.5	144	11.8
4	101	8.0	90	7.4
5	82	6.5	58	4.8
6	59	4.7	30	2.5
7	48	3.8	26	2.1
8	31	2.5	20	1.6
9	24	1.9	17	1.4
10	26	2.1	14	1.1
11	11	⎫	5	⎫
12	12	⎬	5	⎬
13	8	⎬ 4.3	6	⎬ 2.0
14	7	⎬	0	⎬
15	13	⎭	9	⎭
16-20	23	1.8	11	0.9
21-25	20	1.6	8	0.7
26-30	12	0.9	5	0.4
31-50	22	1.7	4	0.3
>50	9	0.7	3	0.2
Total	1257	100.0	1219	100.0
Mean partners*	6.20		3.90	
N/K	32		22	

*Among those with one or more partner (initiated)

This range cannot be interpreted properly without considering variations in the numbers of years of experience of different respondents. Table 9.3 relates the mean numbers of partners to the age bands of the respondents. A graphical representation is given in Figure 9.2. Even this can be misleading (for reasons developed later) but it is sufficient for the moment to note that the accumulated number of partners did not

Table 9.3

Age of Respondent and Total Heterosexual Partners

Males
Total Partners

Age Group (yrs)	0	1	2-3	4-6	7-10	> 10	Total*	Mean**
<19	125	58	86	55	28	17	369	4.65
19-20	40	40	39	36	20	15	190	5.17
21-22	16	13	17	27	10	20	103	8.41
23-24	7	19	11	11	8	12	68	6.49
25-30	13	28	28	34	19	24	146	7.68
31-45	11	49	65	54	26	37	242	7.28
>45	2	43	32	24	12	11	124	4.87
NK	1	3	3	1	6	1	15	7.93
Total*	215	253	281	242	129	127	1257	6.20
(%)	(17.1)	(20.1)	(22.4)	(19.3)	(10.3)	(10.1)	(100)	

Females
Total Partners

Age Group (yrs)	0	1	2-3	4-6	7-10	> 10	Total*	Mean**
<19	99	42	35	12	5	1	194	2.40
19-20	54	38	57	15	12	2	178	2.89
21-22	27	35	37	18	7	8	132	4.18
23-24	11	24	38	18	11	3	105	3.56
25-30	25	56	72	50	14	15	232	4.26
31-45	15	63	96	56	24	23	277	5.09
>45	5	49	30	8	4	4	95	2.78
NK	5	4	1	1	–	–	6	1.83
Total*	236	306	366	178	77	56	1219	3.90
(%)	(19.4)	(25.1)	(30.0)	(14.6)	(6.3)	(4.6)	(100)	

*NK for total partners
**mean partners of initiates only

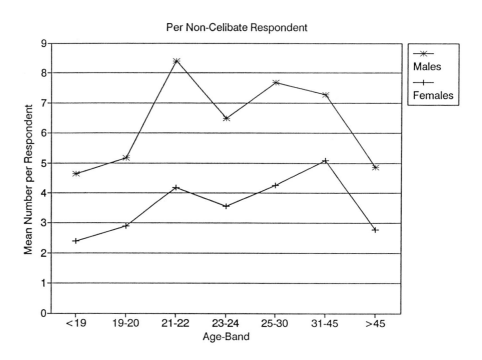

Figure 9.2

Total Heterosexual Partners, by Age

Per Non-Celibate Respondent

increase steadily with increasing age. Both for males and for females the accumulation was irregular, and for the males the total reached a peak and then declined. In terms of personal experience this is of course impossible and it indicates the presence of a cohort effect. The rate of acquisition of new partners was much greater in younger individuals belonging to later cohorts, such that some of these groups had already overtaken the 'final' totals of groups some years their senior. The problem of disentangling the equally powerful effects of age and of birth cohort upon levels of sexual activity, is deferred to a later stage of the analysis.

The Gender Difference

We had hoped to confirm the accuracy of our results by identifying an equality of reporting in male and female respondents. For a large and representative sample from a closed society, observed over a sufficient number of years, the number of new male partners taken by the females, is exactly the same number as the number of new female partners taken by the males. The *rates* of partner acquisition in males and females may not be exactly the same, since this depends also upon the relative numbers of sexually active males and sexually active females sharing the same number of new partnerships. In addition, the frequency distribution and the age distribution of numbers and rates among males and females may differ. But the total **numbers** should be the same, and a check for equality should offer a comment upon veracity. As we have seen, however, there was a wide discrepancy between the numbers reported by the two sexes.

There are several possible interpretations. First, the men may tend to exaggerate and the women to understate their activities. Second, the forms of bias within the sample may differ between the males and females, with the result that the women are not representative of the female partners of the sampled men: nor vice versa. Third, a period of rapid increase in activity between successive cohorts could interact with different age preferences of men and women seeking partners of the opposite sex, to produce a gender difference of this kind. We shall analyse this proposition later. Finally, part of the difference may be taken up by female prostitutes not represented among the females in our sample.

Use of Female Prostitutes by Men

Male respondents were asked whether they had ever had sexual intercourse with a female prostitute; 82 (6.4 percent) said that they had and 1018 (79.0 percent) said that they had not, while the remaining 14.7 percent failed to answer. (This last group consisted mainly of those who had never had sexual intercourse and who treated the question as non-applicable). The 82 men were then asked to say on how many occasions they had had sexual intercourse with a prostitute, within each of several age bands (<19, 19-20, 21-25, 26-30, 31-35, 36-40, 41-45, >45). Altogether, 255 encounters were recorded. This amounted to 4.0 percent of all the heterosexual partnerships reported by the men. The majority of the men who had used prostitutes admitted to only 1 or 2 encounters within individual age bands; 21 men recorded between 3 and 9 encounters within individual age bands; 4 recorded 10 or more.

Those men who had used female prostitutes differed in other aspects of their sexual behaviour, and in their ages. Among the 82 users of prostitutes, 13.4 percent said that they had also had a sexual relationship with a man: compared with only 4.9 percent of those who had not used female prostitutes. The proportions having homosexual anal intercourse, among the users and non-users of prostitutes, were 6.1 percent and 2.1 percent respectively. More of the older men reported the use of prostitutes than did the younger men. Among those up to age 26 at the time of the enquiry, 5.1 percent reported prostitute usage compared with 10.2 percent of those who were aged 27 or more. Part of the gradient is due to accumulated experience, but an especially high level among men of 45 or more (12.0 percent) suggests a cohort effect, with more recent cohorts using prostitutes less.

Homosexual Relationships

The male respondents were asked about sexual relationships with another man. 74 men (6.0 percent of the 1227 who answered the question) said that they had had a sexual experience with another man; and, among them, 44 (3.6 percent of those 1227 answering) said that they had had anal intercourse with another man. Of this last group, 25 (67 percent) had also had sexual intercourse with a woman, while the remainder claimed to have had no sexual intercourse with a woman, only anal intercourse with a man. Most, 20, of the 44 men reporting anal homosexual intercourse had only had one partner; 11 had had two partners; 7 had between three and five partners; and 6 had more than five. The maximum number of partners, reported by one man, was 22. The questionnaire asked about usual style of anal homosexual intercourse. Of the 36 men who answered this, 18 (50 percent) were always or usually the passive (receptive) partner; 8 (22 percent) were always or usually the active (penetrative, insertive) partner; and 10 (28 percent) adopted both roles equally. Respondents were also asked their age at first homosexual intercourse; 21 (58 percent) of the 36 who replied said that this was before the 16th birthday, and 9 of them were before the 13th birthday, down as low as age 6. Some must have been examples of child abuse although we did not ask about this.

Heterosexual Anal Intercourse

We enquired whether respondents had ever had anal intercourse with their heterosexual partners. Among the males, 206 (16.9 percent) of the 1217 who answered the question said that they had; among the females, 171 from among 1200 (14.2 percent). The proportions engaging in heterosexual anal intercourse were fairly constant across the range of ages of our respondents. In contrast with the use of female prostitutes, the proportions above and below age 27 were almost identical, both in men and women.

Initially, the questionnaire did not elaborate further on heterosexual anal intercourse but after discovering that this was a not infrequent practice we amended the questionnaire and included two additional questions. They asked with how many partners the respondent had practised heterosexual anal intercourse, and how often this practice occurred. There were 133 men who said that they had had heterosexual anal intercourse and who were asked the additional questions. Among them, 50.3% had practised it once, 42.3% practised it occasionally and 7.4% regularly; 70.7% had practised it with only one partner, 12.0% with two partners, and 17.3% with 3 or more partners. Among the 110 females who said yes and were asked the subsequent questions, 52.5% had attempted heterosexual anal intercourse only once, 46.7% practised it occasionally, and only one woman regularly; only 7 women said that they had had anal intercourse with more than one of their male partners.

Secondary Indicators of High Risk Sexual Activity

The questionnaire asked about past occurrences of sexually transmitted disease. Among the men, 61 (4.9 percent) of the 1244 who replied said that they had had a venereal disease: and 52 of 1218 women (4.3 percent). 14 of the 61 men and 20 of the 52 women said that they had had gonorrhoea: 5 of the men and 4 of the women had had gonorrhoea more than once. It is possible that some respondents might have had an STD without knowing specifically that it was called gonorrhoea. Both in men and in women the greatest numbers of respondents who had ever had STD's were among those currently aged 27-35.

The women were asked about terminations of pregnancy. Among the 1247 who answered this question, 174 (14.0 percent) had had a termination. The proportion of positive replies increased steadily across the age groups with the exception of the over 45's, as shown in Table 9.4 and in Figure 9.3.(Only those who were sexually initiated are included).

Figure 9.3

Pregnancy Terminations, by Age

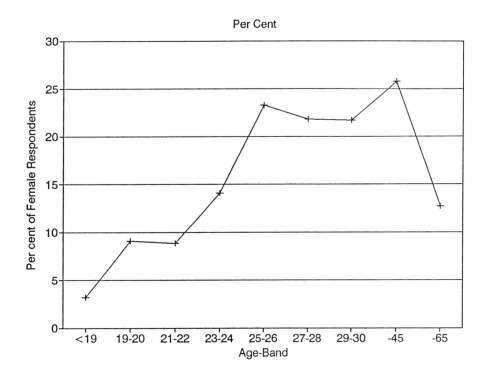

Table 9.4

Frequency of Past abortion: and Age of Female Respondents

	Age Group (yrs)									
	< 19	19-20	21-22	23-24	25-26	27-28	29-30	31-45	> 45	Total*
Abortion	1	10	12	14	21	17	15	69	15	174
No abortion	30	100	123	85	69	61	54	198	103	823
Total	31	110	135	99	90	78	69	267	118	997
(%)	(3.2)	(9.1)	(8.9)	(14.1)	(23.3)	(21.8)	(21.7)	(25.8)	(12.7)	(17.5)

*Includes only initiated females

Figure 9.4

Risk Factors and Social Class

Males

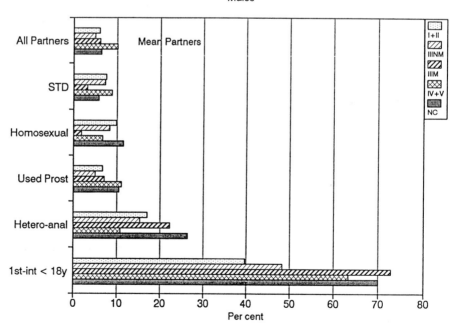

Table 9.5

Sexual behaviour and Social Class

Males (initiated with either sex)	Social Class				
	I & II	IIINM	IIIM	IV & V	Unclassified
No. of cases	225	207	357	49	244
1st heterosexual intercourse <18 years (%)*	39.6	48.3	72.9	63.3	70.0
Total heterosexual partners (mean)*	6.1	5.0	6.2	10.2	6.5
Heterosexual anal sex (%)*	17.1	15.4	22.2	10.9	25.1
Use of prostitute (%)*	6.8	5.0	7.1	11.1	11.7
Homosexual relationship (%)	9.9	8.4	1.8	6.8	11.5
Homosexual anal sex (%)	3.6	3.0	1.2	6.8	7.0
Sexually transmitted disease (%)	7.6	7.4	3.2	8.9	5.9

*Excludes 16 cases initiated with male only

Females (initiated)	Social Class*				
	I & II	IIINM	IIIM	IV & V	Unclassified
No. of cases	296	361	69	47	223
1st heterosexual intercourse <18 years (%)	45.8	48.7	59.4	39.1	55.9
Total heterosexual partners (mean)	4.6	3.7	4.2	3.3	3.3
Heterosexual anal sex (%)	17.1	17.1	10.4	17.4	21.3
Pregnancy termination (%)	19.7	15.4	10.3	23.9	19.6
Sexually transmitted disease (%)	6.4	5.3	2.9	0	5.5

*Based on woman's own occupation

Social Variations in Sexual Behaviour

Variations of sexual behaviour according to social class, ethnic group, age at leaving fulltime education, educational qualifications and marital status are summarised in Tables 9.5 to 9.9. These results relate only to respondents who are sexually initiated, and those who gave no information for a particular question are excluded for that particular item.

Among men, earlier age at first intercourse, the total number of heterosexual partners and the use of prostitutes were all more frequent in the manual social classes (IIIM, IV and V). *(See Table 9.5 and Figure 9.4)*. Heterosexual anal intercourse, the occurrence of sexually transmitted disease, homosexual relationships and homosexual anal intercourse, showed no clear-cut differentiation in these terms.

Among women, neither age at first intercourse, nor pregnancy terminations, nor the practice of heterosexual anal intercourse, were noticeably related to the manual/non-manual dichotomy *(Figure 9.5)*. There was weak evidence of a gradient in the opposite direction, highest in social classes I and II and lowest among social classes IV and V, for the total number of heterosexual partners and the incidence of sexually transmitted disease. Here, however, the numbers of subjects in the lower social classes were small.

Table 9.6 shows ethnic group variations. There were higher proportions of early intercourse, of heterosexual anal intercourse, and a higher use of prostitutes, among the Indo/Pakistani men; but lower proportions of early first intercourse, pregnancy

Figure 9.5

Risk Factors and Social Class

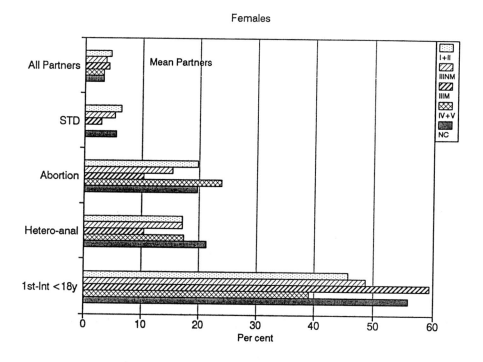

Table 9.6

Sexual behaviour and Ethnic Group

	Ethnic Group			
Males (initiated with either sex)	Cauc	Afro/Car	Ind/Pak	Other
No. of cases*	854	57	129	27
1st heterosexual intercourse <18 years (%)**	58.1	63.2	71.8	65.4
Total heterosexual partners (mean)**	6.3	7.2	5.3	4.6
Heterosexual anal sex (%)**	19.1	12.0	32.2	4.2
Use of prostitute (%)**	6.4	7.3	18.2	11.5
Homosexual relationship (%)	7.4	3.8	7.8	9.1
Homosexual anal sex (%)	3.2	3.8	6.0	9.1
Sexually transmitted disease (%)	5.6	15.1	4.2	4.0

*15 cases excluded NK for ethnic group

**Excludes 16 cases initiated with a male only

	Ethnic Group			
Females (initiated)	Cauc	Afro/Car	Ind/Pak	Other
No. of cases*	769	136	57	31
1st heterosexual intercourse <18 years (%)	51.3	44.4	31.6	69.0
Total heterosexual partners (mean)	4.3	3.2	1.6	2.2
Heterosexual anal sex (%)	18.4	11.5	17.3	26.7
Pregnancy termination (%)	15.9	31.8	11.5	13.3
Sexually transmitted disease (%)	4.5	11.9	1.9	3.3

*3 cases excluded NK for ethnic group

terminations and STD's, and a smaller number of total partners, among the Indo/Pakistani women. Afro-Caribbean men were similar to Caucasians except that they reported higher rates of STD. Pregnancy terminations and STD's were relatively high among the Afro-Caribbean women.

Sexual behaviour in relation to educational qualifications and age of leaving full-time education is shown in Tables 9.7 and 9.8. Men with the highest educational qualifications and those who left full-time education at age 20 or older, had later first

Table 9.7

Sexual behaviour and Educational Qualifications

	Qualification Group			
		Voc/CSE/		
Males (initiated with either sex)	**None**	**'O'-level**	**'A'-level**	**Higher**
No. of cases*	184	568	120	144
1st heterosexual intercourse <18 years (%)**	58.8	68.6	54.7	31.2
Total heterosexual partners (mean)**	7.7	5.8	6.9	5.3
Heterosexual anal sex (%)**	15.6	21.7	27.2	10.7
Use of prostitute (%)**	12.2	6.2	9.6	7.1
Homosexual relationship (%)	4.7	6.4	13.7	9.9
Homosexual anal sex (%)	2.3	3.5	6.8	4.3
Sexually transmitted disease (%)	5.2	4.7	9.3	7.6

*66 cases excluded NK for qualification

**Excludes 16 cases initiated with male only

	Qualification Group			
		Voc/CSE/		
Females (initiated)	**None**	**'O'-level**	**'A'-level**	**Higher**
No. of cases*	129	548	144	125
1st heterosexual intercourse <18 years (%)	39.8	56.4	50.0	32.8
Total heterosexual partners (mean)	3.7	3.9	3.4	5.4
Heterosexual anal sex (%)	16.8	18.6	17.1	16.5
Pregnancy termination (%)	20.0	18.1	17.4	15.6
Sexually transmitted disease (%)	1.6	5.9	5.6	6.5

*50 cases excluded NK for qualification

intercourse, a lower number of total partners and lower rates of heterosexual anal sex. Prostitute usage, and sexually transmitted disease showed no trend. Homosexual anal intercourse was more common among those with A levels or higher qualifications and among those who either left full-time education at older ages or were still there. As with the men, women with higher qualifications and those late in leaving full-time education had later first intercourse. Unlike the men, the total number of partners was highest in

Table 9.8

Sexual behaviour and Age at completing Full Time Education

	Age at completing FTE			
Males (initiated with either sex)	**Still there**	**16 or less**	**17-19**	**20+**
No. of cases*	89	630	254	92
1st heterosexual intercourse <18 years (%)**	79.5	67.7	46.4	27.3
Total heterosexual partners (mean)**	7.5	6.2	6.2	5.3
Heterosexual anal sex (%)**	35.0	19.5	18.9	9.2
Use of prostitute (%)**	9.8	7.3	7.6	9.2
Homosexual relationship (%)	14.1	5.4	6.0	15.4
Homosexual anal sex (%)	10.6	2.9	2.0	5.4
Sexually transmitted disease (%)	2.3	4.8	8.5	7.7

*17 cases excluded NK for age left F.T.E.

**Excludes 16 cases initiated with male only

	Age at completing FTE			
Females (initiated)	**Still there**	**16 or less**	**17-19**	**20+**
No. of cases*	68	494	338	81
1st heterosexual intercourse <18 years (%)	63.2	52.7	49.1	25.0
Total heterosexual partners (mean)	2.9	3.9	3.5	6.4
Heterosexual anal sex (%)	21.5	17.8	16.4	16.3
Pregnancy termination (%)	6.2	17.3	20.6	16.0
Sexually transmitted disease (%)	0.0	5.5	4.5	11.1

*7 cases excluded NK for age left F.T.E.

---

these groups. Pregnancy terminations, except for being low among those still in full-time education, did not vary according to educational indicators. STD's were lowest among those still in FTE and among those with no educational qualifications.

Marital status showed strong relationships with the different sexual behaviour indicators *(Table 9.9)*. The total number of partners was highest among the divorced, separated and widowed groups, for both men and women, although the overall

Table 9.9

Sexual behaviour and Marital Status

Males (initiated with either sex)	Marital Status		
	Single	Married	Div/Sep/Wid
No. of cases*	681	359	38
1st heterosexual intercourse <18 years (%)**	72.9	36.4	56.8
Total heterosexual partners (mean)**	6.1	5.9	11.6
Heterosexual anal sex (%)**	22.2	15.4	21.6
Use of prostitute (%)**	6.6	10.2	8.3
Homosexual relationship (%)	7.9	6.0	10.8
Homosexual anal sex (%)	4.4	1.4	10.8
Sexually transmitted disease (%)	6.3	4.6	11.1

*4 cases excluded NK for marital status

**Excludes 16 cases initiated with male only

Females (initiated)	Marital Status		
	Single	Married	Div/Sep/Wid
No. of cases*	572	325	94
1st heterosexual intercourse <18 years (%)	57.7	35.6	56.0
Total heterosexual partners (mean)	3.8	3.1	7.1
Heterosexual anal sex (%)	18.1	14.2	26.1
Pregnancy termination (%)	14.9	18.4	31.5
Sexually transmitted disease (%)	6.7	3.4	3.2

*5 cases excluded NK for marital status

numbers of respondents in these categories were relatively low. Early first intercourse however was more common among the single respondents, especially the men. Heterosexual anal intercourse was lower among the married groups, both men and women, as were STD's. Homosexual relationships were more common among the divorced/separated/widowed men, this being most marked for homosexual anal intercourse. Among the women, pregnancy terminations were much more common in the divorced/separated/widowed groups.

There were significant inter-correlations among several of the different high risk factors. For example, 11 percent of women who had a pregnancy termination had also had a sexually transmitted disease, compared with 4.0 percent among those who had not had an abortion. Among women who practised anal intercourse with a man 9.9 percent had had an STD compared with 4.0 percent of those who had not practised this form of intercourse. Similarly 11.2 percent of the men who had had heterosexual anal intercourse had had an STD, compared with 3.8 percent of those who had not practised this form of sexual intercourse. Among men who had practised heterosexual anal intercourse with a woman, 9.6 percent had also had a sexual relationship with a man, compared with 5.1 percent of those who had not had heterosexual anal intercourse. And among those men who had reported having a sexual relationship with another man, 21.6 percent had had an STD, compared with only 3.9 percent of those who had only had heterosexual sex. The men who had used prostitutes were more likely to have had anal intercourse with a female (39.2 percent), compared with 17.5 percent of those who had not reported prostitute use. And 21.3 percent of those who had had intercourse with a prostitute, had experienced a sexually transmitted disease, compared with 4.3 percent of those who had not used prostitutes.

Conclusions

The sexual behaviour patterns of both men and women, but especially men, varied according to social class, ethnic group, marital status and educational levels. Many of these variations were concordant with each other, having regard to the demonstrable correlations between the social indicators themselves. Some of these indicators of high risk behaviour were likewise correlated with each other.

However, the pattern of inter-correlation was not entirely concordant, and there was a severe degree of statistical confounding between the different variables. In particular, the social educational and ethnic groupings are each constituted differently in terms of the respondents' ages, their birth cohorts, and their marital status. It would be difficult at this stage to say which of the associations of the different aspects of social behaviour were primary, and which were statistically secondary.

We saw in previous chapters that the sample was socially biased and it now appears that it is relatively short of those social groups with higher levels of sexual activity and the greatest prevalence of high-risk behaviours. Extrapolations from the sample to the population taken as a whole would clearly require some adjustment. However, it would be unwise to carry this analysis further or to attempt any sample-calibration of the behaviour measures displayed, until we have examined how far the behaviour variations are secondary to age and cohort differences in the different social groups.

Chapter 10 – The Quality of Response

This chapter examines the quality and the accuracy of the data supplied by the respondents: especially with respect to the frequencies and patterns of partner-change. There is no way of testing the truthfulness of the responses against external reference points, because there are none. Nor was there any way of testing the repeatability of responses because of the commitment to anonymity. The appraisal therefore depends mainly upon measuring degrees of consistency between responses to different questions with overlapping contents. The questionnaire had been planned from the beginning to make this possible. We also planned to cross-check the stated behaviour of female respondents with respect to their male partners, against that of male respondents with respect to their female partners.

Available Consistency Checks*

The questionnaire was designed to permit correspondence checks between the different parts of different questions. The most straightforward was that between Q15 (total number of heterosexual partners) and Q14 (numbers of new heterosexual partners in each of the successive age bands). Where the Q15 total was less than 16, the exact number was 'ringed'; and it should then be the same as the sum of the categories in Q14. Where the Q15 total was greater than 16, and expressed in the form of a range, the two responses should still be compatible.

In those questionnaires where there were ten or fewer partners, the majority, those listed in Q12 (the latest ten) should also equal those in Q14 and Q15 (above). Individuals listed in Q7 (live-in partners) and Q13 (new partners in the last six calendar years) should always be less than or equal to those recorded in Q12, Q14 and Q15. For young respondents, whose first intercourse was within six years of the date of the enquiry, the total in Q13 should exactly equal the numbers given in Q14 and Q15. Unless there were more than ten partners, it should also equal the number listed in Q12. For male respondents, any incidents of sexual intercourse with prostitutes (Q16) should be included within the corresponding age-band totals in Q14. All these equalities and inequalities were checked.

Date compatibilities were also tested. For example, the dates given for the latest ten partners in Q12 should match dates given in Q13 (numbers of new partners by calendar year) wherever they were within the calendar range of Q13. Entries to Q12

*It will be helpful for the reader to refer to the Questionnaire in Appendix A7 whilst reading this section.

and entries to Q13 should always find an age-matchable entry among the age-banded new partners recorded in Q14. However, Q14 entries matched a corresponding record in Q12 only where there were fewer than eleven partners overall: and in Q13 only where the calendar range was appropriate.

Question Q7, enquiring about live-in partners, including wives and husbands, asked the age at which they first set up common residence, rather than the age at first intercourse. These responses could not therefore be compared exactly with responses in other sections which did ask this question. However, age and date at first intercourse should never have been later than the cohabitation date recorded in Q7. All of these date and age correspondences were checked.

At first, these dating and numerical consistency checks were carried out by direct inspection of the records. Later, as the different kinds of error were identified, computational methods were developed for their recognition.

The Observed Inconsistencies

In fact, there was a wide and varied range of inconsistencies within individual questionnaires; more than sufficient to justify the attention we had given to the problem at the design and analysis stages. There must be doubts about any survey results which omit to take these precautions. Many respondents with complicated sexual careers found it impossible to reduce the components to a questionnaire format. Some of them realized this, and took the trouble to attach explanatory annotations. The least consistent accounts were generally those involving large numbers of partners, and we could not discard these questionnaires without imposing a serious bias upon the activity levels recorded.

At the same time, these records could scarcely be treated as if they were qualitatively homogeneous, so a system was developed for classifying their consistency. We constructed seven classes, ranging from those which were so incomplete as to be unusable (class 1), to fully consistent heterosexual histories (class 6), and unambiguously null histories (class 7). The intermediate classes (5,4,3 and 2) represented increasing levels of inconsistency. Reports in class 5 had a single error whose nature could easily be diagnosed through references to other questions, while class 4 reports showed either two errors which permitted reasonable interpretation, or else a single error which was not easily interpretable. Class 3 reports were less reliable, with more than one error, sometimes partly correctable, but with residual incompatibilities. Class 2 reports were more complex still, usually containing several irreconcilable errors, and sometimes with multiple and gross inconsistencies. The numbers falling within these different classes are displayed in Table 10.1.

Table 10.1

Consistency of Records in Males and Females

Numbers and cumulative percentages (cp)*

Consistency Class	Male number	cp	Female number	cp
1. Incomplete/unusable	43	4.0	33	3.2
2. Multiple errors	199	22.2	99	13.0
3. Several errors, not reconcilable	45	26.4	29	15.8
4. Two errors/partly reconciled	164	41.4	173	32.8
5. Correctable single error	241	63.6	350	67.3
6. Consistent heterosexual history	396	100	333	100
7. Unambiguous null-history	201	–	224	–
Total	1289	–	1241	–
Mean total partners**	6.20		3.90	

*Cumulative percentages (cp) represent proportions of initiated respondents (Classes 1 to 6) and are accumulated row by row from the least reliable of all (Class-1) to Class-6.

**Mean heterosexual partners among initiates.

Components of Inconsistency: Omissions

Some questionnaires lacked fundamental items. For example, 17 males and 6 females failed to give their year of birth; and 16 males and 5 females who claimed to have had sexual intercourse, failed to give their age at first intercourse. In many of these records the missing items were reconstructed (to within a year) from the answers to other questions, but most of them had other serious defects as well. In all but two of them the combination of defects led to a Class 1 designation.

The total number of lifetime partners (Q15) was not stated by 28 male and by 17 female respondents all of whom had elsewhere claimed to have had sexual intercourse. Most of these records were also defective in other respects, although less fundamentally so than those described above. Only four of the 28 males and 1 of the 17 females received a Class 1 designation, but 22 males and 16 females received a 'Class 2'. Many of these Class 2 questionnaires had recorded the numbers of new partners in different age bands (Q14), thus enabling reconstruction of the total number of partners from this alternative source. However, most of them had other errors, and only 2 of the males in this group, and none of the females, were entered to Class 3 or better.

Question 14 (numbers of new partners in different age bands) was left blank by 87 males and 91 females who claimed to have had sexual intercourse. In general, these records contained more information than the records described above, the omissions being less fundamental. Although there were 9 of the males and 6 of the females who did have to be designated as Class 1, and 21 males and 16 females designated as Class 2, there was sufficient redundant information in the remainder to permit a diagnosis and to repair of most of the deficiencies. Among them 57 of the males and 69 of the females were designated as Class 3 or better.

The question asking for details of the last ten heterosexual partners (Q12) was left totally blank by 35 non-celibate males and 48 non-celibate females. These omissions were errors, by definition: but, as with Q14 there was sufficient additional material for the majority to achieve a designation between Class 3 and Class 5.

In contrast with the rather sparse omissions already noted, the question asking for numbers and details of live-in partners (Q7), and the question asking how many new partnerships were established in successive calendar years (Q13) were often left totally blank. No entry to Q7 was made by 551 non-celibate males and 380 non-celibate females and Q13 was left blank by 308 and 348. For these questions, however, the majority of the omissions were legitimate. The blank entries for Q7 reflected the fact that many of the respondents had so far been engaged only in casual sexual encounters, without embarking upon a living arrangement. Reflecting this legitimacy, 326 of the 551 blank male questionnaires, and 236 of the 380 female ones, were designated as fully consistent (Class 6) and only 90 males and 28 females were designated as Class 1 or Class 2. Many of the Q13 omissions reflected the fact that any new partnerships had preceded the date-range of the question. The majority were reasonably consistent (Class 5 or Class 6) and only 68 males and 46 females were designated as unusable (Class 1) or grossly inconsistent (Class 2).

Respondents who entered five 'blanks' for Q7, Q12, Q13, Q14 and Q15 were almost always genuine celibates with an unambiguous null-history (Class-7), although a small number (12 males, 9 females) were designated to Class 1 or Class 2.

Respondents who answered all five questions, or all but one of them, were generally consistent in other respects as well, and most of them designated as Class 5 or Class 6. Among respondents who answered any of the five questions, 21.6 percent of the males and 30.4 percent of the females answered all of them; while another 66.4 percent and 55.2 percent respectively, completed four of the five. In the latter group, most of the single omissions were legitimate. The main interpretation problems were among that minority of respondents (12.0 percent of the males and 14.3 percent of the females) who failed to reply to 2 or 3 or 4 of the five questions. Two-thirds of them (67 percent) were designated as Class 2, or 3 or 4.

Components of Inconsistency: Discrepancies

The omission of a whole question, even two whole questions, often allowed straightforward interpretation and straightforward correction. The totals offered in the other questions – provided they were themselves consistent – could be accepted as the 'truth'. Fortunately, the greater part of the numerical deficiencies encountered within the survey fell within these correctable classes.

However, many responses also displayed other kinds of discrepancies. Although numerically less important than the plain omissions, they generated great difficulties of interpretation. Sometimes, the completed questions which might be used to repair an omitted question, were themselves incompatible. This also sometimes occurred in cases where all the questions had been completed. For example, among 972 males who completed both Q14 (new partners in age bands) and Q15 (total partners), only 686 (70.6 percent) gave identical or compatible totals. Among 902 similar females, only 718 (79.6 percent) gave identical or compatible totals. The discrepancies were reasonably even-handed. For both sexes together, 9.1 percent listed more partners in Q15 than in Q14, while 16.0 percent recorded the reverse. Discrepancies in the Q14/Q15 totals often reflected wider inaccuracies and this showed up in the assignation of consistency classes. While 94.4 percent of those with identical Q14/Q15 counts were assigned to Classes 4, 5 or 6, only 46.4 percent of those showing a Q14/15 difference were designated thus.

The Q14 totals of new partners in successive age bands should always have been greater than or equal to the totals given in Q13 (new partners in successive calendar years): and also those in Q12 (details of the previous ten partners). In fact, the Q14 total was less than the Q13 total in 168 (12.2 percent) of the 1378 records (both sexes) in which both questions were completed. The similar Q12 discrepancy occurred in 140 (13.4 percent) of the 1047 in which both questions were completed.

Some of these discrepancies were presumably due to simple arithmetical errors on the parts of the respondents, but for Q14 there appeared to have been a misinterpretation of the terms used. The meaning of a 'new' partner was explained on the questionnaire and reinforced in the researcher's preliminary oral presentation; yet some respondents interpreted 'new' to mean 'new after the first' or 'new apart from the wife/husband'. In 254 questionnaires the age given for first intercourse was not compatible with any entries in Q14. In 710 questionnaires (with some overlap with the previous discrepancy) the age of first marriage was not compatible with any of the ages for a new partner recorded in Q14. In 109 cases the first spouse was not included among the year-dated partners recorded in Q13, even though the dates of the question spanned the appropriate date.

Some of these non-correspondences may have been due to misidentified dates or ages, but the error was so widespread as to suggest a fundamental misinterpretation of the question. For many, 'new' did not include 'first'. It led us to conclude that wherever the Q14 total was less than the number in a comparable question, then it was usually Q14 which was at fault.

Social Variations of Consistency

The proportion of inconsistent returns increased with the total number of reported partners (Table 10.2). This probably reflects the increased scope for error when reporting complex sequences; but it might also indicate a social correlation. Respondents less able to recall their own behaviours, or to understand questions and to

Table 10.2

Consistency Class (CC) and Total Partners

Males   **Total Partners***

CC	1	2	3	4	5	6-10	11-15	16-20	21-25	26-35	36-50	>50	0 or NR	Total*
2	10	6	10	11	10	41	24	14	14	12	16	5	26	199
3	0	0	2	6	5	20	8	3	0	0	0	0	1	45
4	25	26	30	18	26	32	6	0	0	0	0	0	1	164
5	103	43	25	29	13	25	3	0	0	0	0	0	0	241
6	108	71	60	36	27	63	10	6	6	0	6	3	0	396

Females   **Total Partners***

CC	1	2	3	4	5	6-10	11-15	16-20	21-25	26-35	36-50	>50	0 or NR	Total*
2	7	4	3	9	5	22	8	4	7	5	3	2	20	99
3	0	0	3	2	3	11	10	0	0	0	0	0	0	29
4	33	39	25	28	19	27	2	0	0	0	0	0	0	173
5	150	76	60	31	12	21	0	0	0	0	0	0	0	350
6	105	101	49	20	19	25	6	5	1	0	1	1	0	333

*Based on Q15, or an alternative total from another question

formulate answers, might also be those who take larger numbers of partners. If so, then differences between the social structure of our sample and of the population would bias the record of sexual behaviour. We must therefore examine the three-way relationship between total numbers of partners, accuracy of reporting, and the social circumstances of the respondents.

Gender

The distribution of the questionnaire returns according to consistency class, and according to the gender of the respondent, was given in Table 10.1. The Table also gives cumulative percentages of reliabilities, among the non-null histories. The females returned fewer badly completed questionnaires than did the males; 26.4 percent of males scored a consistency of grade 3 or worse, compared with 15.8 percent of the females. However, the proportion supplying completely consistent histories was similar, even slightly greater in the men: 36.4 percent of the males and 32.7 percent of the females.

Table 10.3

*Consistency and Marital Status**

Numbers and cumulative percentages (cp)*

Consistency Class	Single number	cp	Married number	cp	Div/Sep/Wid number	cp
1	30	2.4	33	4.8	8	5.9
2	138	13.3	129	23.4	30	27.9
3	46	16.9	17	25.9	11	36.0
4	270	38.3	57	34.1	8	41.9
5	80	44.6	433	96.7	77	98.5
6	701	100	23	100	2	100
7	425	–	0	–	0	–
Total	1690	–	692	–	136	–
Mean total***						
partners	5.1		4.6		8.4	

*See Table 10.1

**Both sexes together. Marital status NK excluded.

***Mean heterosexual partners among initiates.

The excess of badly completed returns by the males may be explained in part by the relative complexity of their histories, compared with the female histories. Non-celibate males recorded 6.20 female partners in Q15, on average, while the females reported a mean number of 3.90 male partners. We shall return to the interpretation of the difference itself, later.

Marital Status

Distributions according to marital status are given in Table 10.3. Single respondents were relatively reliable, with only 16.9 percent in Consistency Classes 1 to 3, compared with 25.9 percent among married respondents and 36.0 percent among the divorced and widowed. The more varied partnership histories among those ever married, compared with the singles, probably contributed to these differences.

The 'ever married' were especially liable to the error of misinterpreting the meaning of a 'new' partnership: as described earlier. When we compared the different marital states in terms of Consistency Classes 1 to 4, instead of 1 to 3, the differences between them were much less.

Social Class

The distribution of the Consistency Classes according to the social class of the respondent, is given in Table 10.4. The social classes of the women respondents were based upon their own occupations, rather than those of their husbands.

There was evidence of deteriorating consistency from Social Classes 1 and 2 to Social Classes 4 and 5. The proportions in the Consistency Classes 1 to 3 increased from 15.5 percent to 40.2 percent across this range. The proportion in Consistency Classes 1 to 4 increased from 29.4 percent to 53.6 percent.

Part of this gradient was no doubt due to an increasing unfamiliarity with filling in forms in general, in handling questions, in formulating answers and completing questionnaires. Part, but only part, may be due to an increased intricacy of the sexual histories and an increased mean number of partners in Social Classes IV + V. There was no evident gradient of partner numbers among the women (see Table 9.5). That for the two sexes combined, as shown in Table 10.4, was modest.

Table 10.4

Consistency and Social Class**

Numbers and cumulative percentages (cp)*

Social Class

Consistency Class	I & II		IIINM		IIIM		IV & V	
	number	cp	number	cp	number	cp	number	cp
1	9	1.7	19	3.3	10	2.3	3	3.1
2	58	12.9	54	12.8	87	22.2	27	30.9
3	14	15.5	19	16.1	19	26.6	9	40.2
4	72	29.4	111	35.6	70	42.7	13	53.6
5	211	69.9	197	70.1	76	60.1	26	80.4
6	157	100	171	100	174	100	19	100
7	44	–	90	–	45	–	4	–
Total	565	–	661	–	481	–	101	–
Mean total*** partners	5.2		4.2		5.9		6.8	

*See Table 10.1

**Both sexes together; unclassified excluded.

***Mean heterosexual partners among initiates.

Educational Ages and Qualifications

The respondents were classified according to their educational and vocational qualifications, as shown in Table 10.5. They range (left to right) from those with no qualifications at all, or none recorded, through those with vocational or CSE qualifications, GCE 'O' levels, or GCE 'A' levels to diplomas/degrees. There was a marked difference between the first group and the remaining groups with respect to the proportions in Consistency Classes 1 to 2, or 1 to 3, or 1 to 4. There was less difference, although a consistent trend, across the remaining 4 educational groups. For example, 39.3 percent of those with no qualifications were designated as Class 3 or worse: descending through 22.3 percent, 16.0 percent, 15.0 percent and 14.2 percent in the more qualified groups. This gradient was associated among men with greater numbers of partners: a mean of 7.7 among the unqualified, descending to 5.3 among those with diplomas or degrees (See Table 9.7). Among the women, the gradient of mean numbers of partners ran counter to the educational gradient, a point to which we return later.

Table 10.5

*Consistency and Educational Qualifications***

Numbers and cumulative percentages (cp)*

Qualification Group

Consistency Class	None Recorded number	cp	Vocational/ CSE number	cp	'O'level number	cp	'A' level number	cp	Higher number	cp
1	30	6.7	8	3.4	22	2.5	7	2.6	9	3.3
2	127	35.3	39	19.7	84	12.0	25	12.0	23	11.7
3	18	39.3	6	22.3	35	16.0	8	15.0	7	14.2
4	70	55.1	42	39.9	149	32.9	39	29.7	37	27.7
5	123	82.7	66	67.6	213	57.0	70	56.0	119	71.2
6	77	100	77	100	379	100	117	100	79	100
7	73	–	36	–	220	–	69	–	27	–
Total	518	–	274	–	1102	–	335	–	301	–
Mean total partners***	5.7		4.6		4.9		4.9		5.3	

*See Table 10.1

**Both sexes together. Qualification NK excluded.

***Mean heterosexual partners among initiates.

Table 10.6

Consistency and Ethnic Group**

Numbers and cumulative percentages (cp)*

| | Males | | | | | | Females | | | | | |
| | Cauc | | Afro/Car | | Ind/Pak | | Cauc | | Afro/Car | | Ind/Pak | |
CC	number	cp	number	cp	number	cp	number	cp	number	cp	number	cp
1	20	2.4	4	6.6	8	6.2	19	2.4	4	2.9	7	10.9
2	144	19.3	19	37.7	27	27.3	72	11.7	17	15.2	5	18.8
3	34	23.3	4	44.3	5	31.2	26	15.0	3	17.4	0	18.8
4	125	38.0	9	59.0	24	50.0	116	29.9	38	44.9	12	37.5
5	217	63.5	5	67.2	13	60.2	298	68.3	26	63.8	19	67.2
6	311	100	20	100	51	100	247	100	50	100	21	100
7	103	–	10	–	76	–	64	–	52	–	93	–
Total	954	–	71	–	204	–	842	–	190	–	157	–
Mean total partners***	6.3		7.2		5.3		4.3		3.2		1.6	

*See Table 10.1

**Other ethnic groups and ethnic group NK excluded.

***Mean heterosexual partners among initiates.

Ethnic Group

The consistency distribution is shown in Table 10.6 for Caucasians, Afro/Caribbeans and Indo/Pakistanis, separately. Males are shown in the left-hand panel and females in the right-hand panel. Separate demonstrations for the two sexes were necessary because the ethnic distributions within our sample were different for males and for females.

The Table shows that the proportions of inconsistent records were greater among the Afro/Caribbean and Indo/Pakistani groups than they were among the Caucasians. This was so both for males and females although more marked for the males. Among the females the Afro/Caribbeans and Indo/Pakistanis were similar; but among the males, the Afro/Caribbeans were less consistent than the Indo/Pakistanis. The gender difference in reliability noted earlier was present within each of the ethnic groups. That is, the ethnic and gender differences appeared as independent phenomena; neither was secondary to the other.

There was no clear relationship, here, between levels of inconsistency and mean numbers of partners. The consistency differences should probably be attributed to differences in language skills.

Conclusions

This chapter has demonstrated the great difficulties which many respondents had in returning reliable and consistent records. Reliability varied systematically according to their educational, social class and ethnic groups and according to the complexities of the sexual histories which they were trying to record. The social variations were themselves correlated with complex histories. It is reasonable to suppose that the errors arose for both reasons: the varying difficulty of the task, and varied abilities to remember the relatively distant past, to add up, to understand questions, and to formulate answers.

However, this cannot explain the difference between the numbers of partners reported by the male and female respondents. The females were generally better at filling forms than were the males. The difference must stem from other factors. The first is probably a sampling problem arising from selection through the work place. The females selected in this way were not representative of the partners of the males within the sample: nor vice versa. This included an absence of prostitutes among the women in the sample. It is possible also that the males tended to exaggerate some of their answers, while the females were more reticent. Finally, as we show later, there was an interaction between rapid cohort changes in sexual activities in recent years and the offset age preferences of males and females seeking partners.

From the pragmatic point of view of analysing the material we had to decide whether to ignore the errors and use the discrepant records as they stood: or to omit the least satisfactory records from our analyses: or to try to repair some of the errors. For some returns there was no choice; they could not be analysed and had to be omitted. For the others, however, it was clear that the least satisfactory records were also the most complex, involving greater numbers of partners, so that their omission would seriously bias the results among the remainder. For them there was no option but to 'correct' the discrepancies using the planned redundancy of the data. This process is described in the next chapter.

Chapter 11 – Interpreting Sexual Histories

As we have described in detail in Chapter 10, many sexual histories were inconsistent or incomplete. The level of inconsistency varied, sometimes to the point of fragmentation, and a few returns were so chaotic or incomplete as to be unusable. The most frequent errors were omissions. Sometimes a whole question was omitted; sometimes one part of a complex question. The record of a single partnership might be missing, or sometimes a detail such as the calendar date of first contact, the duration of the relationship, the frequency of intercourse, the use of condoms . . . and so on.

The likelihood of an inconsistency or omission increased with the complexity and intricacy of the recorded behaviour, and with the total number of sexual partners. There was no satisfactory solution to be had from simply omitting inconsistent records since this would have introduced serious selective bias to the remaining fraction of the sample. The redundancies designed into the questionnaire were therefore used to repair the defects to the degree that was possible. The remainder of this chapter provides a detailed technical description of the method used to achieve this. The reader wishing to follow this sequence, at this stage, will need to refer constantly to the questionnaire forms displayed in the Appendix to Chapter 7. For other readers it may be sufficient to read only the conclusions to the present chapter before proceeding to Chapter 12.

The basic technique was to identify each partner according to the recorded details, to search for parallel records of the same partner in other questions, and to delete duplicates while counting the first record. To be technically exact, the duplicates were disqualified by adding a temporary marker, rather than physically deleted. The most effective ordering of the process was developed by printing out the successive steps and comparing them visually with the original record. The algorithm was developed in stages until the differences between the computer and visual approaches were as small as could be managed.

Each identified partner was 'counted' into a matrix whose columns and rows represented the year of birth of the respondent and the age at which the identified sexual partnerships began. The sequence eventually adopted for assembling the 'counting matrix' was as follows.

The identification sequence

Use of Prostitutes

The first step in the process was to exclude a potential arithmetic inconsistency relating to the use of prostitutes. Q14 had asked for the numbers of new partnerships undertaken in successive age bands, and respondents were also asked to include one night stands and other short relationships, as well as longer-term partners. Male respondents were also asked in a different question (Q16) whether they had ever had sexual intercourse with a prostitute: and if they had, then how many times this had occurred at different ages, the age-bands being in the same format as in Q14. If both questions were correctly answered, then the numbers given in Q16 should also have been included in Q14.

There was a possible ambiguity in that Q14 asked for the *onsets* of new partnerships, while Q16 asked for individual *acts* of sexual intercourse with a prostitute. A regular client of a single prostitute might legitimately have entered greater numbers to Q16 than were included in Q14. However, few respondents had used prostitutes regularly and we found no examples of returns which suggested that the heavy users tended to visit particular prostitutes. For the purposes of analysis, each prostitute contact was treated as a 'new' partnership. It was supposed that whenever the Q16 response was less than or equal to the Q14 response, the prostitute encounters had been correctly incorporated in Q14; but when the Q16 response exceeded the Q14 response, the Q14 value was enlarged to contain that given in Q16. Records of prostitute encounters duplicated in Q14 were thus deleted, but any remaining prostitute encounters were added to the respondent's Q14 record.

Age at First Intercourse

Following the elimination of the above arithmetical problems, the identification sequence proper began with the identification of the first partner. Age at first intercourse was recorded in Q11. This event was treated as the first entry to the respondent's 'counting matrix'. A search was then made for the earliest record in the age-banded Q14, and if a matching age was found it was treated as duplicate of the Q11 entry, and removed. Age at first intercourse was also converted to calendar year at first intercourse by referring to year of birth. A search was then conducted in each of Q7, Q12 and Q13 for the calendar year of the earliest recorded partner and this was also tested against the year derived from Q11. Again, if a match were obtained, the duplicate record was removed.

The initial stage of these calendar-year searches permitted a latitude of plus or minus one year around the calculated calendar year of first intercourse. However, as soon as a first correspondence was detected, the year was considered 'fixed', and the tolerance allowed in comparing dates in subsequent questions was eliminated. The purpose of this manoeuvre was to avoid deleting a record in error, where two separate records were each compatible with the first intercourse record, but incompatible with each other.

Marriages and Live-in partners

Q7 was scanned for undeleted partners with whom the respondent had lived. Each partner was added to the 'counting matrix' and duplicates were then sought in Q12, Q13 and Q14. The mechanism was similar to that followed for first intercourse except that the primary item of information recorded was the calendar year and it was the corresponding age (with a designated latitude) which had to be calculated.

The partners in Q7 were sought out and dealt with in four separate stages. In each of these stages the full set of Q7 entries were scanned. The first stage sought non-marital partnerships whose durations were less than a year. In these partnerships, the date given for first cohabitation could be accepted as the date of first intercourse and compared with the dates of first intercourse recorded in Q12 and Q13. This scan of Q7 – like later scans – was carried out in reverse order, beginning with the most recent entries. This follows the supposition that the more recent entries would be best remembered and most accurately recorded.

The second and third stages sought out marriages. Q7 was scanned to find the date of the first marriage – strictly, the year in which the respondent started living with his/her first spouse. 'Living with' does not necessarily correspond with the year of first intercourse with a spouse, as asked in Q12 and Q13, or the age at first sexual intercourse as asked in Q14. Where no exact match was found, a reasonable match with an earlier date was sought, and this was then deleted. In a few cases deleted entries may not in fact have been duplicates. In the third stage, later marriages were scanned in a similar way. Finally, live-in partnerships which did not fall within any of these previous classes, were examined.

In each of these four stages the identified Q7 partner was entered to the counting matrix, and duplicates in later questions were deleted.

The Last Ten Partners

Q12 had asked about the last ten women/men with whom the respondent had sexual intercourse, identifying the calendar year of first intercourse. The remaining entries in Q12, those which had not already been deleted because they matched entries in earlier questions, were next entered in turn to the counting matrix and a search carried out for duplications in Q13 (calendar year of new partners) and Q14 (age band of new partnerships). Once more, duplicate entries were deleted.

New Partners in the Last Six Calendar Years

The format of Q13 varied at different stages of the survey, accommodating different sequences of dates. However, the form of the question remained constant. The questionnaire asked for numbers – and not for identifying details as in Q12 – of new partnerships undertaken in particular calendar years. Each partner recorded in Q13 should have been matchable with a remaining non-deleted entry in Q14. Where a corresponding entry in Q14 was in fact found, it was deleted. However, although a Q13 entry should always be found in Q14, the reverse did not necessarily apply. An early age-band partner in Q14 might have been acquired in a calendar year preceding the range of Q13. It was for this reason that the scanning of Q14 was left until last.

Residual Identities

The final stage identified the residual entries in Q14 – those which had not been deleted on the grounds of correspondence with records of partners in earlier questions. These residual identities were then eligible for entry to the age/year-of-birth counting matrix. In some cases, however, there was a problem.

Some records had residual entries in more than one place, partners identified in earlier questions who could not be located – as they should have been located – in Q14. For example, there may have been a partner in Q12 who could not be found in Q14: and yet a partner in Q14, left over at the end, who had not been identified anywhere else. The process therefore retained a tally of earlier 'residuals' to set against the Q14 residuals at this later stage.

In situations such as this there were two possibilities. Either there were indeed two separate partners, each recorded in one of the two questions and omitted in error from the other: or else the details of year and age of a single partner had been entered inconsistently so that the rules of identification had failed to associate the one record with the other.

Visual inspection of the records suggested that most of these discrepancies were of the second type, and this could often be confirmed in the computational sequence, by comparing the total number of identified partners with the total number recorded by the respondent in Q15. If the duplication turned out to have arisen from misidentification, then we had to ask whether the dating of the first or the second of the mis-specified partnerships was correct.

A computational device was adopted in which both of the suspect records were entered to the counting matrix in order to contribute to the form of the age/cohort distribution; but the total number of partners was 'scored' as the mean of those separately identified, and the respondent's own stated total. This was taken to be the greater of the number given in Q15, and the sum of those given in Q14. Meanwhile, a running total was kept, for all respondents, of a) the totals estimated through individual identification, and b) the greater of the numbers recorded in Q14 and Q15. When the matrix for the total group was finally assembled, it was recalibrated to provide values corresponding with the midpoint of these two grand totals.

Individual differences between the numeric total and the total of 'identified' partners were sometimes positive and sometimes negative and when it came to assembling population sub-groups they partly cancelled out. The calibration factors which had to be applied to the group counting matrix were therefore modest. The numerical totals were generally less than the sums of the separate identifications. The ratio was usually close to 1.0, but ranged from 0.86 to 1.03.

Calculating the Rates

The events assembled into the cohort/age-band matrix served – after calibration – as the numerators for subsequent calculations of rates of partner-change. The denominators to these rates consisted of a similarly constructed matrix of the number of person years of opportunity which each individual contributed to the total group experience. This denominator matrix had the same structure as the numerator matrix and its content was assembled in parallel with the numerator assembly. For each respondent the year of birth was identified and, within this column of the matrix, the rows corresponding with all ages from 14 onwards, and less than the correspondent's current age, were incremented by one year of experience. For the current age, the increment was taken to be 0.5 years.

The rates of partner change at different ages and in different birth cohorts were calculated by dividing one matrix by the other. The results are described in the next chapter.

Conclusions

The sexual histories exhibited a wide variety of inconsistencies, but there was usually sufficient redundant information to correct them. An algorithmic sequence was developed, and evaluated through visual cross-checks between the printed steps of the process, and the original records. The basic technique was to assemble a count of individually identified partners, omitting duplicate records, and checking it against the numeric totals in answers to other questions. The first of these estimates tended to exceed the second and, for purposes of assembling group statistics, the mid-point was chosen, and a corresponding calibration factor applied to the aggregated age-cohort matrix of identified partnerships.

Chapter 12 – The Acquisition of New Partners

Chapter 11 described how the numbers of years at risk (the denominators) and the numbers of new partners acquired (the numerators) were assembled into the columns and rows of a matrix representing the birth year of the respondent and his/her age at the start of the partnership. The years and ages were subsequently blocked into quinquennial (or sometimes finer) groups. Annual rates of new-partner acquisition were then calculated for each birth cohort and age group. This was also done separately for the different social and demographic groupings.

This complex procedure was designed to eliminate the effects of age and cohort variations between compared sub-populations. Age and birth-cohort proved to be among the most powerful of the sexual behaviour determinants, and different sub-groups in our sample differed in these terms. For example, Table 9.6 of Chapter 9 shows that Afro/Caribbean males recorded an average of 7.2 sexual partners, compared with 6.3 among Caucasian males. Might this represent a true difference in behaviour patterns? Alternatively, did the groups differ in respect of the numbers of years for which they were 'exposed', or did they differ with respect to their age distributions or the birth-cohorts to which they belonged? When their experiences were corrected for the numbers of person years of experience, the two groups were closely comparable, with 44.8 partners per hundred years of experience for the Caucasian males, and 43.6 for the Afro/Caribbean males. But even this does not answer all the questions.

Overall Rates of Partner Acquisition

Table 12.1 gives the results of dividing the partner-acquisition matrix by the years-of-experience matrix. The result is expressed as the mean number of new partners per 100 years of experience between the 15th birthday and the date of the enquiry. The later birth cohorts (the right-hand columns of the Tables) were truncated at relatively early ages, while the earlier-born cohorts (the left-hand columns) supplied histories covering a much wider age span.

The right-hand totals of Table 12.1 give age-band means across all cohorts, and show that the most active partner-acquisitions occurred in the youngest age groups. After a small reduction between the first and second age-bands in both males and females, there was a steep subsequent decline in the rate at which partners were acquired. The totals at the foot of each panel represent the mean partner acquisition rates for separate cohorts, summed across the available age bands. These totals show a steady increase in

Table 12.1

Partner acquisition rates per 100 Years of Experience

Quinquennial birth cohorts and 5-year age-bands

Three main ethnic groups combined

Male Respondents

Age at partner acquisition	Quinquennium of birth							
	1940-5	1946-9	1950-4	1955-9	1960-4	1965-9	1970-6	Total
15-19	40.63	44.63	73.71	63.64	43.30	73.40	95.56	69.81
20-24	25.28	40.66	34.95	37.46	66.23	110.3		57.52
25-29	14.38	25.71	24.71	27.90	56.73			30.04
30-34	8.29	13.98	20.89	26.10				16.26
35-39	4.50	15.53	18.31					11.49
40-44	5.39	12.12						8.01
45-49	7.61							7.30
All ages	17.30	26.67	37.34	41.30	54.11	85.33	97.70	46.50

Based on 6449 new partners and 13869 person-years of experience at age 15 or greater

Female Respondents

Age at partner acquisition	Quinquennium of birth							
	1940-5	1946-9	1950-4	1955-9	1960-4	1965-9	1970-6	Total
15-19	14.91	20.83	30.07	38.61	30.29	40.30	44.74	35.00
20-24	13.58	17.99	20.35	25.95	34.77	49.18		31.13
25-29	7.00	11.39	10.56	22.01	26.30			16.94
30-34	3.12	8.08	12.18	15.69				10.07
35-39	3.37	17.26	15.43					11.49
40-44	2.42	19.95						8.11
45-49	4.29							4.21
All ages	6.91	15.75	18.45	27.33	31.10	43.07	45.87	25.20

Based on 3766 new partners and 14946 person-years of experience at age 15 or greater the rate of acquiring partners from the 1940-1945 cohort towards the 1970-1976 cohort.

The steepness of the negative and positive slopes in these two sets of marginal totals is deceptive, because the distributions within the body of the Table are not independent of each other. The later age groups are overloaded with early cohorts, and the later cohorts are overloaded with young respondents. However, the gradients in the marginal totals are each present within individual rows and columns of the Table as well. These separate trends, less steep than the marginal trends, supply a more valid representation of behaviour changes with age and with cohort, than do the aggregated ratios.

Table 12.1 indicates changes according to calendar periods, as well as according to age and birth cohort. Calendar quinquennia are represented by diagonals – south west to north east. For example, activities at age 15-19 among males born 1955-59 (63.64 in the Table) represent a calendar period surrounding the year 1974. The values 34.95, 25.71 and 8.29, following the same diagonal, are contemporaneous, and the summed activities between ages 15 and 34, in a notional calendar quinquennium centred upon 1974, amounted to a mean of 33.2 new partners per 100 years of experience. The rate in the preceding quinquennium was similar. The comparable rates for the following calendar quinquennia were 29.8, 47.1 and 72.2. Among females, the successive rates from 1974 onwards were 18.4, 18.7, 27.3 and 34.0. These upward calendar trends accord with general experience, although the rapid acceleration in the later cohorts, and in the calendar period from 1984 onwards, are perhaps surprising. This is the period corresponding with the AIDS pandemic and with large-scale publicity warning of the dangers of promiscuous behaviour.

The rates in Table 12.1 can also be assembled to show cumulative numbers of partners acquired by different ages. The results for the separate quinquennial birth cohorts, males and females, are shown in Figures 12.1 and 12.2. The increments are shown, here, in 5-year steps and the vertical columns of the two figures, in which the various cohorts overlap, represent calendar quinquennia. The secondary X-scale on the figures indicates the calendar quinquennia in which the increments took place. These rates are the genuine cumulative values, unlike the cross-sectional accumulations shown earlier in Table 9.3. The figures show that all cohorts continued to accumulate partners for as long as they were followed, but the pace of accumulation increased from one cohort to the next. The earliest cohort (born in 1940-45) accumulated partners at a relatively rapid pace up to age 25 and at a much slower pace after age 30. The next cohort, born in 1946-49 started in the same way, but at a rate which soon overtook the 1940-45 cohort. By age 25, both males and females had acquired more partners than the earlier cohort had acquired by age 30. The 1950-1954 cohort likewise overhauled the 1946-49 cohort by the time they were 25, and the preceding cohort had reached 30. This pattern continued, with each new curve equalling or surpassing the curve of earlier

Figure 12.1

Cumulative Sexual Partners of Males

Birth-Cohorts : by Age

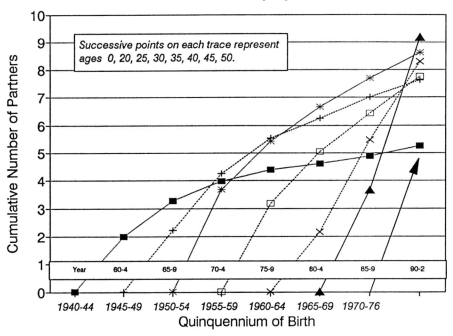

cohorts. The initial slopes became steeper and steeper, and the slowing down with age progressively attenuated. These overlapping cumulative cohort assemblies indicate the levels which completed partnership tallies may reach. They show how mid-career interception by the survey itself has truncated the final numbers.

Social and Demographic Variations

Table 12.2 gives overall partner acquisition rates according to ethnic group, social class, educational level, marital status and age of first intercourse. As well as the simple overall rates per 100 years of experience, Table 12.2 supplies a Standardised Acquisition Ratio (SAR), analogous with a Standardised Mortality Ratio (SMR). This is the ratio between the observed number of partners in a sub-group and the number which would have been expected if the demographic structure of the sub-group had been the same as that in all the sub-groups put together. Specifically, the expected number is calculated by multiplying aggregate partner-acquisition rates in each age

Figure 12.2

Cumulative Sexual Partners of Females

Birth-Cohorts : by Age

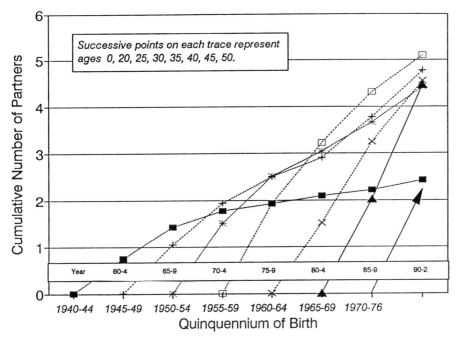

and cohort division by the numbers at risk, in these divisions, within the sub-group to be standardised. The components are added together and the sum is compared with the sub-group total.

Some of the associations already described survived the standardization process, or were even enhanced; but not all. The most striking modification is shown in the first panel of Table 12.2 which shows that the standardised ethnic variation is the inverse of that which the simple count of partners (Table 9.6) had suggested. The Caucasians now showed the greatest standardised acquisition rates both for males and for females. The Indo/Pakistani males showed a higher rate than the Afro/Caribbean males, while the Indo/Pakistani females showed a lower rate than the Afro/Caribbean females. Because the ethnic differences would have complicated the subsequent analyses displayed in Table 12.2, the remaining paragraphs of the Table refer to Caucasians only.

There was a distinct social class gradient in SAR among the Caucasian males, but not among the females. In this examination, the females were classified by their own occupations, rather than their husbands' or partners' occupations. Variations of the

Table 12.2

Partner acquisition rates per 100 Years of Experience: Standardized Ratios*

	Males		Females	
	Rates	SAR	Rates	SAR
Main Ethnic Groups	46.5	100.0	25.2	100.0
Ethnic Groups				
Caucasian	44.8	102.4	25.9	111.0
Afro/Car	43.6	79.6	26.0	81.9
Indo/Pak	60.7	95.3	15.9	45.8
Social Class (Caucasian)				
I+II	35.5	88.3	28.5	108.0
IIINM+IIIM	45.2	92.1	25.9	94.0
IV+V	52.9	112.6	21.1	104.1
Marital Status (Caucasian)				
Single	74.1	100.3	42.1	107.2
Married	28.1	93.4	14.2	72.6
D/Sep.	58.8	176.8	28.1	148.3
Widowed	50.5	128.3	31.4	168.7
Educational Qualification (Caucasian)				
Nil	36.3	127.4	14.1	92.5
CSE/vocational	46.7	99.1	25.3	98.1
GCE: O,A	62.3	105.3	30.3	100.6
Diploma/degree	36.2	75.5	31.6	103.3
Age of leaving F.T.E. (Caucasian)**				
0-15 years	32.1	122.9	14.2	101.9
16-18 years	54.0	100.7	28.3	94.8
19-20 years	40.7	83.5	25.3	77.9
21 or more	31.0	64.2	42.0	150.7
Age at first intercourse (Caucasian)				
-19 years	122.2	210.8	63.0	184.3
20-24 years	52.1	104.5	34.7	111.0
25-29 years	24.9	59.8	16.5	72.6
30 or more	7.1	21.0	7.8	41.3

*The Standardized Acquisition Ratio (SAR) is the ratio between the observed and expected number of partners: multiplied by 100. The expected numbers in each paragraph of the Table are based upon the products, within each cell of the age-cohort matrix, of the years of experience of the sub-group and the specific rate of acquisition for the aggregate.

**Including those still in full-time education at current ages within these bands.

SAR according to marital status conformed with variations of the simple rates (see Table 9.9). Married men and married women showed lower SAR's than did those still single, or those who were divorced or separated or widowed. The differences in crude rates were diminished by standardisation, reflecting the excess among the singles of those who were young and belonged to later cohorts. However, the difference was still present and probably does represent a genuinely reduced level of partner-change among those who marry and stay married. The pattern was similar for both sexes.

Panels 4 and 5 of Table 12.2 examine the effects of the two indices of educational level: the attainment of formal qualifications, and age on terminating full-time education. The SAR for the men displayed a clear gradient according to the latter. Those who left school early showed twice the SAR of those who continued their education beyond the age of 20 years. The finding was reflected in their educational qualifications. Those obtaining degrees or diplomas displayed half the SAR of those who had no qualifications at all.

The educational gradients in the females however were paradoxical. The SAR rose according to the level of qualification obtained, instead of falling, and was greatest among those obtaining diplomas or degrees. The age at leaving full-time education in women, showed the same initial trend as that observed in the men: but it then reversed, so that the highest rates of all were in those continuing their education to the age of 21 or beyond. While further education was sexually inhibiting for the males: it seemed to be sexually liberating for the females. However, the true interpretation may not be so direct. There may be additional reasons for these differences. Levels of education, sexual activity and occupation may have interacted in such a way as to determine selective entry to – or exclusion from – our sample.

The last panel of Table 12.2 shows gross variations of crude partner acquisition rates, among non-celibates, according to the age at first intercourse. The standardisation process ameliorated somewhat the extreme differences between the earliest and latest ages but there was still a very steep gradient. There was a four-fold difference of extremes among the females and a ten-fold difference among the males. The differences were much greater than the lead-time of the early start itself could have explained. Subsidiary analyses showed that there were steep gradients for the rates of partners acquired *after* the age of 20, according to the earliness or lateness of the first partnership *before* the age of 20. At the earliest first-intercourse ages, variation by a single year had a remarkable effect upon later behaviour. This is illustrated in Tables 12.3 and 12.4.

For example, men born in 1950-54 and having first intercourse at 15 years of age or earlier, had accumulated an average of 30 partners by the age of 40. Men in the same cohort and having first intercourse just one year later, at 16 years of age, accumulated only 14.1. Similarly, men starting intercourse at 17 years accumulated 10.9; and men

Table 12.3

Cumulative Numbers of Heterosexual Partners:

Age at First Intercourse in Males

Birth Cohorts

First intercourse at 15 years of age or less

By age	1940-4	1945-9	1950-4	1955-9	1960-4	1965-9	1970-6
20	11.6	9.9	17.5	12.4	10.7	12.6	11.6
25	13.4	13.5	23.0	16.4	20.8	21.3	
30	15.7	16.4	27.1	17.3	25.7		
40	17.2	20.6	30.0				
50	17.9						

First intercourse at 16 years of age

By age	1940-4	1945-9	1950-4	1955-9	1960-4	1965-9	1970-6
20	5.4	7.0	9.3	8.5	5.4	6.3	5.1
25	7.4	9.1	10.6	10.5	8.6	14.2	
30	8.4	9.6	11.5	13.9	15.0		
40	9.3	11.0	14.1				
50	10.2						

First intercourse at 17 years of age

By age	1940-4	1945-9	1950-4	1955-9	1960-4	1965-9	1970-6
20	4.5	4.5	6.8	4.2	3.9	4.8	5.2
25	5.3	10.6	8.2	5.0	7.4	11.0	
30	5.4	14.1	10.3	6.0	10.1		
40	5.7	15.8	10.9				
50	6.7						

First intercourse at 18 years of age or later*

By age	1940-4	1945-9	1950-4	1955-9	1960-4	1965-9	1970-6
20	1.2	2.4	2.0	1.8	2.5	2.6	4.0
25	2.7	4.3	3.7	3.7	5.2	6.4	
30	3.3	5.4	5.1	4.9	6.9		
40	3.7	6.5					
50	3.9						

*Includes those having passed this age, and not having had sexual intercourse at the time of enquiry

Table 12.4

Cumulative Numbers of Heterosexual Partners:

Age at First Intercourse in Females

Birth Cohorts

First intercourse at 15 years of age or less

	1940-4	1945-9	1950-4	1955-9	1960-4	1965-9	1970-6
By age							
20	2.3	8.3	3.9	7.2	5.8	7.3	7.5
25	3.3	11.2	4.6	8.7	10.6	10.8	
30	3.8	11.5	5.5	10.6	13.4		
40	4.5	15.5	7.7				
50	5.0						

First intercourse at 16 years of age

	1940-4	1945-9	1950-4	1955-9	1960-4	1965-9	1970-6
By age							
20	3.3	3.7	3.4	4.2	4.9	5.3	6.2
25	4.2	4.9	4.8	5.5	6.5	8.8	
30	4.7	5.3	5.4	7.3	8.2		
40	5.3	8.5	7.7				
50	6.1						

First intercourse at 17 years of age

	1940-4	1945-9	1950-4	1955-9	1960-4	1965-9	1970-6
By age							
20	2.4	2.8	4.6	3.9	3.2	4.0	5.3
25	2.9	3.4	6.9	5.4	5.2	5.8	
30	3.7	4.0	7.0	6.5	7.0		
40	4.6	5.6	9.2				
50	4.6						

First intercourse at 18 years of age or later*

	1940-4	1945-9	1950-4	1955-9	1960-4	1965-9	1970-6
By age							
20	1.3	1.3	2.2	2.9	1.8	2.5	3.8
25	2.5	2.6	3.6	4.9	4.0	5.4	
30	3.0	3.3	4.4	6.0	5.4		
40	3.2	4.2	5.8				
50	3.6						

*Includes those having passed this age, and not having had sexual intercourse at the time of enquiry starting at 18 years of age or later, only 5.1. The pattern was less regular among the females, but still evident.

These variations possibly reflect individual differences in the skills of acquiring partners, but more probably an environment with widely varying levels of opportunity and peer-pressure. Alternatively – or additionally – initial success may disperse inhibition, develop technique or increase desire.

Age at First Intercourse

Whatever the mechanism of the above associations, age at first intercourse clearly serves as an extremely powerful predictor of subsequent sexual behaviour. Its associations are more powerful than for any other variable examined. It is clearly not an indirect effect of these other factors, whether alone or in combination. It reflects a high

Figure 12.3

Cumulative Sexual Initiations of Males

Birth-Cohorts : proportions by Age

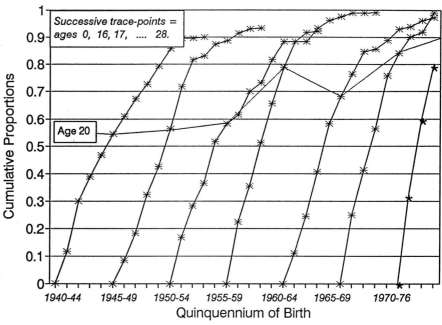

degree of individual variation *within* each of the different social and occupational/ educational strata.

The distribution of ages at first intercourse was displayed in Table 9.1 but took no account of the non-uniformity of the sample, which contained decreasing numbers with increasing age. Table 12.5 and Figure 12.3 correct for this bias. They supply a better picture of rates of acquisition, and cumulative acquisition, of first partners.

Figures 12.3 and 12.4 separate the curve of cumulative acquisition of first partners, as given in Table 12.5, into separate curves: one for each birth cohort. Both for men and for women, the cumulative curves tended to get steeper in successive cohorts, although the pattern was not entirely regular. For example, the 1955-59 male cohort was especially vigorous and the following cohort less so. The first three cohorts achieved around a 50 percent sexual initiation by age 20; while the last two cohorts had reached 70 percent initiation by ages 19 and 18 respectively. The women passed the 50 percent mark at ages 20, 20, 19, 18, 19, 18 and 17.

Figure 12.4

Cumulative Sexual Initiations, Females

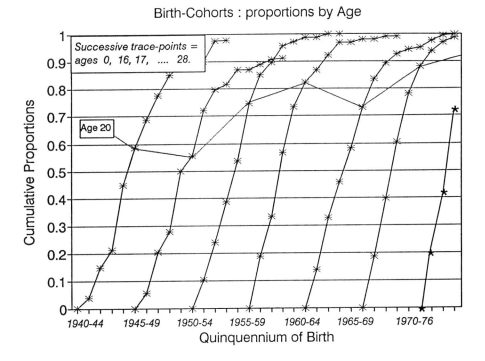

Birth-Cohorts : proportions by Age

Table 12.5

Age at first Intercourse:

Percentage and Cumulative Percentage Distributions

Age	Males		Females	
	percent	cumulative	percent	cumulative
≤16	22.0	22.0	12.9	12.9
-17	17.5	39.5	15.9	28.8
-18	13.5	52.9	17.3	46.1
-19	13.0	65.9	17.4	63.5
-20	8.8	74.8	10.9	74.4
-21	7.1	81.8	8.5	82.9
-22	4.8	86.6	6.0	88.9
-23	3.2	89.9	3.9	92.8
-24	3.8	93.7	1.7	94.6
-25	3.4	97.0	1.4	95.9
-26	1.4	98.5	1.1	97.1
-27	1.1	99.6	2.8	99.8
>27	0.4	100.0	0.2	100.0

The calculated annual values accumulated to more than 100 first partners per 100 experience years: 106.9 for the males and 100.9 for the females. This was due to annual discontinuities in the curve of decline of the population at risk, with increasing age. The percentage and cumulative percentage distributions were therefore adjusted to 100.0

The accelerating rates of sexual initiation and of total partner-acquisitions, both in men and in women, may well explain contemporary increases in cervical intraepithelial neoplasia (CIN). It also explains the long known fact that cervical cancer is associated with early age at first intercourse. It has commonly been supposed that early intercourse was harmful per se, but the powerful relationship between it and the total number of partners, as now demonstrated, shows that the first serves as a powerful proxy for the second. The frequency of partner-change, rather than the earliness of first intercourse, is probably the true determining factor. These findings confirm those of other workers (12,13,14,15,16) whose enquiries of the antecedent sexual experiences of women with cervical pathologies have demonstrated that the association with early age of first intercourse was secondary to an association with the total number of partners.

The rapid increases in partner acquisitions, in recent years and in recent cohorts, offers a partial explanation of the different sexual histories of the men and the women in our sample. Records of marriages and maternities show that male partners tend to be older than their female partners by about five years. The female partners are from more recent birth cohorts than their male consorts. A cross-sectional sample such as our own therefore selects women from earlier cohorts than those who are the female partners of the sampled males. We should therefore expect parity between males and females in cohorts separated by about five years. The effect can be seen by comparing curves from male and female cohorts in Figures 12.1 and 12.2 which are offset by one quinquennium. Relating the first three cumulative points of the 1960-64 male cohorts, and the first three points of the 1965-69 female cohorts, eliminates much of the crude gender difference.

Standardised initiation ratios (SIR) were calculated in the same way as the SAR's in Table 12.2. In general, social and demographic variations of initiations were less striking than those for total acquisitions. There was still a moderate social class gradient for males, but not for females. The most striking differences between SAR's and SIR's related to educational qualifications and the age at leaving full-time education. Neither of these factors showed any effect upon SIR, either in males or in females. It would appear that educational factors influence only the subsequent partner-acquisitions, rather than initiations.

However, there were clear relationships between early age at first intercourse and other indicators of promiscuity. Among the 43 men recording a sexually transmitted disease 89 percent had already had first intercourse by age 19, as had 92 percent of the 34 women with STD. The 103 women reporting a termination of pregnancy had reached 90 percent sexual initiation by age 19. Of the 33 men – among the heterosexually initiated – who admitted to having had anal intercourse with a man, 79 percent had achieved their heterosexual initiation by the age of 19 years.

Residual Variations

Although much of the overall variation in the total number of partners was explained by the different mean values in different birth cohorts and according to ages at first intercourse or the different social variables: there was a major degree of residual variability *within* each of the sub-groups. The distributions of numbers of partners within the different sub-strata were always wide and highly skewed. The variances of the distributions were far wider than the calculable 'random' values represented in a poisson distribution. This was confirmed by the chi-square tests for dispersion *within* the different strata, which were highly significant. There is therefore ample evidence that individual variations of behaviour, within the sub-groups, are as important as the effects of the group differences themselves.

Conclusions

The varying age and cohort structures of the different sub-sets of our sample demanded a sophisticated form of analysis in which age-annual and calendar-annual events were accumulated jointly; converted then into partner acquisition rates; and finally into indirectly standardised indices of activity for each separate sub-group. This form of analysis was conducted separately for first sexual partners, as well as for all partners.

Many of the social and demographic associations demonstrated in the crude tabulations of Chapter 9, survived standardization. As in the crude tabulations there was a pronounced gradient, in Caucasian men, according to social class, according to education qualifications and according to age at leaving full-time education. In women, the social class effect was absent and the educational effects were reversed. The social class effects were present both for first partners and for subsequent partners, but the educational effects related almost entirely to subsequent partners. Married persons of both sexes had had fewer partners than the singles, or the divorced or separated. The most striking reversal of an initial finding based upon crude counting related to ethnic group. Standardized acquisition rates were now greater among Caucasians than among Afro/Caribbeans or Indo/Pakistanis.

Apart from the powerful effects of age and of birth cohort, the most striking new finding was the striking effect of early age at first intercourse upon the total number of subsequent partners. This was found both among males and among females. This appeared to be a primary association, not statistically secondary to the social and demographic variations. It has important subsidiary implications with respect to the etiology of cancer of the cervix.

The distribution of the total numbers of partners within the whole sample was highly skewed, with a high variance. Part of the variation could be attributed to the social and demographic stratifications, and to the effect of age at first intercourse: but not all of it. There remained a substantial degree of individual variation within each of these sub-groups, far beyond anything which could be attributed to a random sampling effect.

The combined demonstrations of the social variations of overall activity, and the social biases of the sample, suggest that our group was numerically deficient with respect to the most sexually active classes. Calculations of sexual activities based on our sample must therefore under-represent those in the population at large. The extent of this under-representation cannot be calculated directly but is probably epidemiologically significant. Population levels of activity could be about 1.5 times greater than those demonstrated.

Chapter 13 – Age Relationships

The age-preferences of those seeking new sexual partners affect the spread of a chronic sexually transmitted infection. A close correlation between the ages of the partners will limit diffusion between age groups. It will ensure that senior cohorts, having attained an increased prevalence with increasing age and opportunity, will remain relatively isolated from the following cohorts. They will grow older and withdraw progressively from partner-change activity; and those with AIDS will die without having transmitted their HIV infections to younger people. However, if the choice of partner is less restricted, providing for abundant cross-contacts between different birth cohorts, then the infection can 'burn-back' from the more highly infected upper age groups of one cohort, to the younger age bands of a following cohort. For the disease to survive, the rate of burn back must be greater than the rate at which current prevalence levels are carried forward to later ages through the aging process.

The annual reports of the Office of Population Censuses and Surveys (OPCS) supply national statistics on the relative ages of partners at marriage and at maternity. They are based upon marriage certificates and birth certificates. However they do not (and can not) supply ages at the beginnings of relationships where the partners neither married nor produced children. The present survey recorded this information. Table 13.1 shows the relationship between the contact ages of our male respondents, against the stated ages of their female partners; while Table 13.2 shows the contact ages of our female respondents, set against the stated ages of their male partners.

Both Tables show a moderately high level of correlation with r = + 0.64 for the male respondents and r = + 0.68 for the female respondents. A combined calculation based upon the pooled data from male and female respondents gave similar results. These values are similar to those found in marriage and in maternity statistics.

These Tables demonstrate 'regression towards the mean'. Young respondents, male or female, were usually paired with the same age or older partners, and older respondents were more often than not paired with younger ones. The pattern differed somewhat in the men and the women, probably because of differences in the ways the male and female samples were obtained. We discuss this in a later chapter. However, the proportions with wide age separations were in each case modest, as the correlation coefficient would suggest. Only 4.1 percent of males under the age of 20 had partnered women over the age of 25. For female respondents the proportion was a little higher, but only 14.1 percent. This will clearly limit the rate at which an infection could diffuse between the age bands.

Surprisingly, our data did not demonstrate the difference between the means of respondents and their partners which available national statistics would lead us to

Table 13.1

Ages of male respondents and female partners

Age of male respondents (x)	Age of female partners (y)										Totals
	-17	18, 19	20, 21	22, 23	24, 25	26-30	31-35	36-40	41-45	46-70	
-17	264	135	39	6	3	6	5	1	1	2	462
18, 19	95	235	99	26	28	17	5	1	2	0	508
20, 21	27	146	141	42	22	23	9	4	1	0	415
22, 23	5	47	93	73	25	21	8	1	1	1	275
24, 25	2	28	47	53	39	35	8	2	0	1	225
26-30	3	13	41	45	50	73	25	10	3	2	265
31-35	0	5	6	11	6	24	18	11	6	2	89
36-40	0	4	4	5	6	8	7	10	3	0	47
41-45	0	0	2	1	1	1	3	5	1	1	15
46-70	0	0	0	0	1	2	0	3	5	3	14

Total partnerships 2305

mean x = 20.81 years

mean y = 20.63 years

$y = 7.68 + 0.62 x$

$x = 7.12 + 0.66 y$

$r = +0.64$

Ages are those given or calculated for the start of those relationships for which sufficient information was supplied. This Table is limited to initiated Caucasians

Table 13.2

Ages of female respondents and male partners

Age of female respondents (x)	Age of male partners (y)										Totals
	-17	18, 19	20, 21	22, 23	24, 25	26-30	31-35	36-40	41-45	46-70	
-17	71	144	75	25	19	15	3	1	2	0	355
18, 19	10	102	107	83	49	57	15	2	5	2	432
20, 21	1	20	74	98	64	67	12	10	1	0	347
22, 23	0	5	27	45	56	73	19	4	3	1	233
24, 25	0	0	11	23	32	59	19	10	5	1	160
26-30	0	3	8	19	27	94	53	25	14	8	251
31-35	0	0	2	9	6	20	27	13	11	10	98
36-40	0	0	1	1	2	11	17	15	10	6	63
41-45	0	0	0	0	0	0	2	5	8	6	21
46-70	0	0	0	0	0	1	1	0	1	5	8

Total partnerships 1968

mean x = 21.30 years

mean y = 24.31 years

$y = 7.15 + 0.81 x$

$x = 7.18 + 0.58 y$

$r = +0.68$

Ages are those given or calculated for the start of those relationships for which sufficient information was supplied. This Table is limited to initiated Caucasians expect. The mean age at the start of a partnership was 20.8 years for male respondents and 20.6 years for their partners. For the female respondents, the mean stated age at the start of a partnership was 21.1 years, and the mean stated age of their partners was only 3 years greater. This is probably the result of sample age-biases, and particularly the relative youth of our respondents compared with the national population, combined with the regression effect.

It is difficult to judge the reliability of these data. Our respondents may not always have known the true ages of their partners. This could have introduced systematic bias if the female partners of male respondents had represented themselves as younger than they really were, or the male partners of the female respondents had represented themselves as older. Alternatively, the respondents may have guessed or retranslated their partners' ages in order to comply with their views as to what was appropriate.

There was one notable discrepancy between the data for the men and the data for the women, which may partly be explained in this way, but which has an important implication. Although men under 18 claimed to have partnered large numbers of women also under the age of 18: women under 18 had far fewer contacts with this age group among their partners. We must conclude that women under 18 who had partners under 18 must have been excluded, very largely, from our sample. The reasons for this are discussed further in a later chapter.

Conclusions

Our data confirm the presence of a moderately high partner-age correlation at the onset of new partnerships, of the same order as that observed among marriages and maternities. This is probably sufficient to restrict the spread of sexually transmitted infections between age bands. The absence of a major age differential between the partners in the sample, when we know that this exists in other circumstances, is probably a sample artefact arising from a combination of regression towards the mean and a non-representative age distribution. The sample exhibited a notable deficiency of young women with young male partners. This must reflect the manner in which the sample was chosen. It will have important implications for our subsequent analyses.

Chapter 14 – Variations on the Partnership Theme

Durations of Partnerships

Respondents were asked how long individually identified sexual relationships had lasted and whether they were now terminated. This information was limited to the maximum of six cohabiting partners recorded in Q7, and the ten latest partners recorded in Q12. Q7 recorded the first year and the duration of the living-arrangement: while Q12 used the date of first sexual intercourse as the start point.

Although it was often possible to equate partners listed in Q7 with those listed in Q12, or to tell them apart, ambiguities sometimes arose from the coarse specification of the dates and durations. As described in Chapter 10, many reports were incomplete, lacking some of the details requested. In the end, interpretable data on durations were extracted from 2412 male-reported and 1885 female-reported separate partnerships. Among these male-reported partnerships, 20.3 percent, and 29.3 percent of the female-reported partnerships, were still continuing. Distributions of the durations for males and females separately, up to their terminations or to the present time, are displayed in Table 14.1.

Overall, the distributions of the durations were wide and bimodal. The two largest classes were a) transient partnerships consisting either of one act of intercourse, or a single-night relationship, or more than one night over a period of less than one month; and b) continuing partnerships which had so far lasted more than 4 years. There were some differences between the men and the women. Relative to the men, the women showed an excess of terminated long-lasting partnerships, and fewer continuing partnerships of short duration. Once more, this suggests that the sampling biases affecting the females were different from those affecting the males.

Mean durations of partnerships were calculated by attaching mid-range values to the terminated partnerships and by supposing that continuing partnerships had been intercepted and recorded halfway through their durations. On this basis the mean duration of the male-recorded partnerships was 1.66 years; and of the female-recorded partnerships, 2.62 years.

The reciprocal of the mean duration in males was 0.60, supplying an alternative estimate of the annual rate of partner change. It corresponds reasonably well with the directly calculated estimate of 0.53. For the females, the reciprocal of 2.62 is 0.38, corresponding exactly with the directly calculated 0.38. These values suggest that

Table 14.1

Durations of Individually Identified Heterosexual Partnerships

Male Respondents

a) Terminated partnerships

Duration to termination in months

duration	1nt.	<1m	1m	2	3	4	5	6	-9	-12	-18	-24	-30	-36	-48	>48	Total
number	564	231	129	139	151	72	33	145	64	118	57	84	11	41	27	57	1923

b) Continuing partnerships

Duration to date in months

duration	-12	-24	-36	-48	>48	Total
number	105	45	52	33	254	489

Total durations=48059 months.   Mean duration in years=1.66
Reciprocal of mean   =0.60

Table 14.1 cont.

Female Respondents

a) Terminated partnerships

Duration to termination in months

duration	1nt.	<1m	1m	2	3	4	5	6	-9	-12	-18	-24	-30	-36	-48	>48	Total
number	239	65	62	78	131	50	25	127	46	133	56	105	23	42	37	114	1333

b) Continuing partnerships

Duration to date in months

duration	-12	-24	-36	-48	>48	Total
number	81	69	53	54	295	552

Total durations=59284 months. Mean duration in years=2.62

Reciprocal of mean =0.38

terminated partnerships had either been followed immediately by another, or had been separated from the next by only a short interval. If some individual partnerships had overlapped, then they were balanced by the intervening intervals in others. These correspondences corroborate the partner-number gender differences already noted. They are not simply a function of exaggeration by the males and reticence by the females. They demand a real explanation.

There is however scope for bias according to duration, among the partnerships for which information was given. The male partnerships in Table 14.1 represent 40.3 percent of all partnerships counted; and the female partnerships represent 48.5 percent. There must have been selective exclusion of transient partnerships among some of those respondents whose records exceeded the capacity of Q12, (details of last 10 partners) or whose sexual careers were too complex to summarise. The true mean durations for all partnerships may be less than calculated; and the rates of partner-change possibly greater.

Frequency of Intercourse

For partnerships recorded in Q12, respondents were asked on how many occasions they had sexual intercourse during the course of each month. The distribution is shown in Table 14.2. This question was not appropriate to that large group of partnerships which lasted for one night only, although some respondents did enter a number: (up to 15!). For the remaining partnerships the detailed distribution was bimodal. The exact form of the distribution was affected by number preferences but there was a first peak at 2-4 times per month, and a second one around 15 times per month. It was this which lead us to select the frequency bands shown in Table 14.2.

This bimodality was present both for men and for women. It was less obvious among the continuing partnerships, where the second of the two peaks predominated, to the near-exclusion of the first. The first peak was especially associated with partnerships lasting less than 6 months as shown in Table 14.2, which combines both terminated and continuing partnerships.

The question had arisen whether very short partnerships carry a disproportionately high risk of HIV transmission: for two plausible reasons. First, a promiscuous sub-culture will probably accommodate a high prevalence of infectives, both for HIV and for other sexually transmitted disease; and second, vigorous partner-switching suggests vigorous personal relationships, and a high frequency of sexual intercourse. This would support an image of recurrent enthusiastic 'honeymoons' with each new partner.

Table 14.2

Frequency of Intercourse and Duration of Partnership

Male Respondents

Duration of Partnership to termination or to date

Monthly Frequency	≤3m*	≤6m	≤12m	≤24m	≤48m	>48m	Total
1-4	368	95	83	44	45	78	713
5-9	127	54	60	43	33	75	392
10-20	134	86	91	87	76	124	598
over 20	17	8	17	8	7	9	66

Female Respondents

Duration of Partnership to termination or to date

Monthly Frequency	≤3m*	≤6m	≤12m	≤24m	≤48m	>48m	Total
1-4	227	86	87	61	50	96	607
5-9	32	53	58	62	56	131	392
10-20	29	53	98	96	92	152	520
over 20	1	4	12	7	8	8	40

*excluding one-night relationships and those of duration ≤1m giving frequency as once per month. Those with frequency not recorded are excluded.

On this last surmise, the data suggest otherwise. Short relationships had an excess of low intercourse-frequencies and a shortage of high ones. For example among men in partnerships lasting up to 3 months, 23.4 percent reported a frequency of intercourse of 10 or more per month, compared with 52.2 percent among partnerships lasting 1-2 years. For women the comparable proportions were 10.4 percent and 45.6 percent. (Table 14.2). We must suppose that many short relationships were established in difficult circumstances which made frequent intercourse difficult; or that they were such casual arrangements that they did not call for it; or that low intercourse frequencies are a mark of those less than satisfactory relationships which are soon abandoned. Whatever the mechanism, these paradoxical associations are likely to ameliorate rather than to aggravate the transmission risks invoked by high rates of partner change.

Exclusivity and Overlap of Partnership

The reported durations of partnerships corresponded with those expected on the basis of the partner-change statistics. *On average*, one partnership followed immediately upon the last. However, these overall statistics could mask a mixed pattern in which some partnerships overlapped while others were separated by gaps. We therefore tried to assess directly the proportion of sexual partnerships where the respondent had undertaken a fresh relationship, before the first one had been abandoned. Not all such events could be detected from our records because of the limited resolution of the given dates. It was impossible to say whether a partnership undertaken during one calendar year, or at a particular age, had started before or after the termination of a previous one in the same year. A limited examination was therefore carried out of those Q7-recorded cohabiting partnerships, including marriages, whose limits (including current limits) were recorded: and those non-corresponding partnerships recorded in Q12 (the latest ten partners) whose onsets were dated, to see how many of the latter had clearly started during the course of the former.

Records of 289 cohabiting partnerships, 134 of which were marriages, were identified among the Caucasian males, where sufficient information was supplied. There were also 370 sufficiently documented cohabiting partnerships recorded by the Caucasian females, of which 192 were marriages. The patterns of intercurrent relationships taking place during the course of the partnerships, and undertaken by the respondents themselves, are given in Table 14.3. There was, of course, no information on activities undertaken by the partners. Both for males and for females the proportions of marriages in which the respondents indicated external partnerships, were greater than for the non-marriage cohabitations; 25.6 percent versus 16.4 percent for the males: and 19.2 percent versus 15.6 percent for the females.

These differences of proportions, as it turned out, were related to the longer durations of the marriages, compared with non-marriage cohabiting partnerships. This supplied a greater duration of opportunity for infidelity. It also enhanced the technical possibility of detecting intercurrent relationships because of inexact reporting (in Q12 and Q7) of the beginning and endings of relationships. For example a partnership which began and ended in the same year or in adjacent years offered no possibility of detecting an intercurrent partnership. The mean duration of reported marriages among the men – measured to their termination or to the date of the enquiry – was 4.5 years, compared with 1.9 years for the non-marriages. For the females the respective durations were 6.3 years and 2.5 years. When this was taken into account, the duration-adjusted rates of intercurrency were greater among the non-marriages than among the marriages. For the males, the marriage intercurrency rate was 14.2 per 100 years of exposure, and for the non-marriages it was 22.0 per 100 years: (22 percent per annum). For the females, the respective rates were 4.4 and 10.1 per 100 years of exposure. Some of these

Table 14.3

Cohabiting Partnerships and Intercurrent Sexual Encounters

Male Respondents

	Number of intercurrent partnerships						
	0	**1**	**2**	**3**	**4**	**≥5**	**Total**
Marriages	215	34	20	6	4	10	289
Non-marriages	115	11	3	2	3	3	134

	Mean duration (y)	**Number of Interlopers**	**Percent Interloped**	**Interloped per 100 yrs.**
Marriages	4.5	184	25.6	14.2
Non-marriages	1.9	55	16.4	22.0

Female Respondents

	Number of intercurrent partnerships						
	0	**1**	**2**	**3**	**4**	**≥5**	**Total**
Marriages	299	56	9	4	0	2	370
Non-marriages	162	23	4	1	0	2	192

	Mean duration (y)	**Number of Interlopers**	**Percent Interloped**	**Interloped per 100 yrs.**
Marriages	6.3	104	19.2	4.4
Non-marriages	2.5	48	15.6	10.1

---

observations may have resulted from dating errors: just as dating errors must have hidden others.

Because the possibility of 'detecting' intercurrent partnerships was hindered by the coarse resolutions of the recorded dates and ages, these findings must be regarded as minima. In addition, the proportions and rates refer to the behaviour of only one of the two partners. The true rates of interloped partnerships must be greater than our material indicates.

Use of Condoms

We asked about the use of condoms within the last ten partnerships (Q12). The four permitted descriptions of condom usage were 'always', 'usually', 'sometimes' and 'never'. As with other questions, the terms and scope of the enquiry were sometimes misunderstood; for 23 male partnerships consisting of a single night, the respondent returned 'sometimes'. It could of course be true.

Table 14.4 shows the proportions of male and female respondents who reported the use of condoms; and it relates these proportions to the durations of the partnerships. As with Tables 14.1 to 14.3 the results are limited to those male and female partnerships for which the reported details reached a sufficient standard. Different respondents omitted different items, and the total numbers given in these Tables, and in later Tables, are not necessarily the same. Indeed, none of the Tables in this chapter is a proper subset of any of the others.

Table 14.4 shows that regular condom usuage was more frequent among the terminated relationships, than for the longer and continuing relationships. This was so for both sexes, although males reported condom usage more often than did the females. This must reflect different selection biases for the two sexes; or else it is a manifestation of the offset-age/cohort interaction discussed earlier; or perhaps a gender-specific reporting-bias. Among male respondents engaged in partnerships which had since terminated, 32.7 percent used them always/usually. The lowest usages were among partnerships which had lasted more than two years. For both sexes together, 18.8 percent of them always or usually used a condom. Because short partnerships imply high switching rates, these condom-usage patterns must ameliorate the enhanced risks born by those with large numbers of partners.

Table 14.5 shows the distribution of condom usage according to the frequency of intercourse. Usages were greater in partnerships with low monthly frequencies. Among males engaging in now discontinued partnerships with frequencies of intercourse up to eight times per month, 36.6 percent used condoms always or usually, compared with 26.1 percent in partnerships with higher intercourse-frequencies. This difference was also observed among the females, but to a lesser degree. Here, 28.5 percent of the partnerships with lower intercourse frequencies used condoms always or usually, compared with 22.8 percent in partnerships declaring higher frequencies.

Table 14.4

Use of condoms and Durations of Partnerships

Males

Terminated Partnerships   **Durations of Partnerships**

Use of condoms	1nt	≤1m	2m	3m	≤6m	≤1y	≤2y	>2y	Total*	%
always/usually	177	146	58	53	96	64	46	23	663	32.7
sometimes	23	38	16	20	41	40	39	49	266	13.1
never	352	256	68	83	121	88	61	68	1097	54.1

Continuing Partnerships   **Durations of Partnerships in years**

Use of condoms	-1	-2	-3	-4	over 4	Total*	%
always/usually	43	14	13	7	58	135	27.1
sometimes	28	19	15	15	100	177	35.6
never	37	12	24	12	101	186	37.3

Females

Terminated Partnerships   **Durations of Partnerships**

Use of condoms	1nt	≤1m	2m	3m	≤6m	≤1y	≤2y	>2y	Total*	%
always/usually	65	59	33	39	60	48	41	30	375	26.1
sometimes	0	13	8	20	32	35	43	79	230	16.0
never	175	82	42	80	123	114	87	131	834	58.0

Continuing Partnerships   **Durations of Partnerships in years**

Use of condoms	-1	-2	-3	-4	over 4	Total*	%
always/usually	22	23	8	12	61	126	22.8
sometimes	23	20	19	12	92	166	30.1
never	36	26	26	30	142	260	47.1

*'not recorded' are excluded. The exclusion criteria are different from those in Tables 14.1 and 14.2 and the row and column totals are not exactly the same. Neither Table is a subset of the other.

Table 14.5

Use of condoms and Frequency of Intercourse

Males

Terminated Partnerships Frequency of Intercourse per month

Use of condoms	-2	-4	-6	-8	-10	-15	-20	>20	Total
Always/Usually	116	83	42	37	26	44	18	8	374
Sometimes/never	167	159	97	59	78	81	83	30	754
Total	283	242	139	96	104	125	101	38	1128
% used	(41.0)	(34.3)	(30.2)	(38.5)	(25.0)	(35.2)	(17.8)	(21.1)	(33.2)

Continuing Partnerships Frequency of Intercourse per month

Use of condoms	-2	-4	-6	-8	-10	-15	-20	>20	Total
Always/Usually	17	18	8	15	17	23	9	3	110
Sometimes/never	23	33	28	29	46	55	41	19	274
Total	40	51	36	44	63	78	50	22	384
% used	(42.5)	(35.3)	(22.2)	(34.1)	(27.0)	(29.5)	(18.0)	(13.6)	(28.6)

Females

Terminated Partnerships Frequency of Intercourse per month

Use of condoms	-2	-4	-6	-8	-10	-15	-20	>20	Total
Always/Usually	66	65	29	19	20	26	16	4	245
Sometimes/never	146	161	81	60	88	83	34	18	671
Total	212	226	110	79	108	109	50	22	916
% used	(31.1)	(28.8)	(26.4)	(24.1)	(18.5)	(23.9)	(32.0)	(18.2)	(26.7)

Continuing Partnerships Frequency of Intercourse per month

Use of condoms	-2	-4	-6	-8	-10	-15	-20	>20	Total
Always/Usually	6	14	15	17	14	9	8	4	87
Sometimes/never	26	34	52	42	54	54	43	14	319
Total	32	48	67	59	68	63	51	18	406
% used	(18.8)	(29.2)	(22.4)	(28.8)	(20.6)	(14.3)	(15.7)	(22.2)	(21.4)

Table 14.6

Condom Usage and Year of Partnership

Males   **Start of Partnership**

Use of condoms	1960-79	1980-84	1985	1986	1987	1988	1989	1990-	Total
Always/Usually	40	43	26	29	56	102	136	176	608
Sometimes/Never	159	206	85	95	140	159	219	202	1265
Total	199	238	111	124	196	361	355	378	1873
% used	(20.1)	(18.1)	(23.4)	(23.4)	(28.6)	(28.2)	(38.3)	(46.6)	(32.5)

Females   **Start of Partnership**

Use of condoms	1960-79	1980-84	1985	1986	1987	1988	1989	1990-	Total
Always/Usually	22	53	25	38	46	54	70	54	362
Sometimes/Never	138	269	106	137	131	99	127	48	1055
Total	160	322	131	175	177	153	197	102	1417
% used	(13.8)	(16.5)	(19.1)	(21.7)	(26.0)	(35.2)	(35.5)	(52.9)	(25.5)

The most striking source of variation for condom usage was related to the calendar years of partnerships as shown in Table 14.6. Usage by males increased from around 20 percent for partnerships starting in the period 1960-1984, through 30 percent in 1988 to 38.3 percent in 1989 and to 46.6 percent in 1990 and 1991. The picture was similar in the females where always/usually usage stayed below 20 percent until after 1985. It had reached 35 percent by 1988 and 53 percent in 1990-91. Overall, the male and female sequences matched well, in contrast with the various gender differences noted earlier. This is probably a calendar-based trend rather than a cohort-based phenomenon, and is less susceptible to gender bias through an interaction between differential age preferences and the cohort trend in switching activity. In addition, females who use condoms are more likely to be selected *into* the sample, rather than excluded through early pregnancies.

Conclusions

This chapter displays some of the ways in which the sexual partnerships varied. They exhibited varied durations, different frequencies of intercourse, different patterns of exclusivity and overlap, and different patterns of condom usage. Each form of variation is statistically related to each of the others. Together, these phenomena add to the problem of constructing a realistic yet technically manageable simulation model for the spread of an infection. However, some of them modify the effects of others such that some of the predictive problems are eased. For example, the disease-transmitting effects of high rates of partner-change were ameliorated by the low frequencies of sexual intercourse and by the high proportion of condom usage associated with high switching-rates. The increasing trend of partner-change in recent years was partly counteracted by an increase in the use of condoms. The gaps and the overlaps between successive partnerships appeared to 'balance' in that the reciprocal relationship between durations of partnerships and rates of partner change, overall, corresponded with those which would have occurred if each partnership had followed immediately after the previous one. All these points must be brought to bear upon the design and operation of a predictive model.

Chapter 15 – Sexual Behaviour: A Synthesis of the Data

It is time now to construct a composite picture of sexual behaviour in our society. The purpose of this chapter is to characterize the pattern of sexual activities within which the HIV epidemic is developing. The first important point is that it is a changing picture: a picture indeed of accelerating change. This is evident both within our own and in other sets of data. The changes include reduced early marriage rates, increased divorce rates, earlier first heterosexual intercourse, increased early pregnancies, increased illegitimate deliveries and a high and accelerating rate of partner-switching. The most significant changes have occurred during the last decade and seem to be continuing.

This raises very serious problems for predicting the future of the HIV epidemic. Against that purpose we are concerned less with the last decade of sexual behaviour than with the next, and with longer term changes beyond. It is necessary to project the changing patterns already observed into the time period for which the HIV predictions are themselves relevant. That is, we shall have to model the changes in the social substrate before we can model the epidemic which grows upon it. Clearly, the technical problems and the uncertainties go far beyond those of sampling bias and responder-consistency, as discussed in earlier chapters.

Sexual Initiation

The data on age at first intercourse were probably reliable. Few non-celibate respondents failed to reply, and the age was probably well remembered. Initiations were affected rather less by social class and educational level than were acquisitions of later partners and so there was less scope for any social or demographic sampling bias. The basic distribution of initiations was given in Table 12.5.

However this form of presentation is insufficiently developed for entry to a dynamic model. A new format shown in Table 15.1 now takes account of numbers of individuals still uninitiated at each age, correcting not only for the age-bias in our sample, but also for the progressive attenuation of those still 'eligible'. It gives age-specific rates of initiation among the remaining non-initiated fraction of the population. It is based on the latest three cohorts, 1960-64, 1965-69 and 1970-76. It shows that the rate of initiation per annum continued to rise with age, at least up to 22 years, with no evidence of a residual reluctant group. Our numbers were insufficient to make any firm

Table 15.1

Sexual Initiation* and Age:

rates/per annum per 100 non-initiated

Age last birthday	Males	Females
15**	31.6	15.7
16	32.2	23.1
17, 18	39.0	31.2
19, 20	44.5	40.3
21, 22	44.1	39.4
23 or more ***	(78.4)	(56.3)

*for individuals born in 1960 or later

**including any initiations before the 15th birthday

***approximate rates based on small numbers

comments much beyond that age. As with the crude figures, the males in this sample outpaced the females.

These results, combined with the evidence of an accelerating rate of initiation (see Figures 12.3 and 12.4) provide an indication of the pattern for the future. We should probably anticipate 50 percent sexual initiation by the age of 17 in males and age 18 in females: and around 90 percent initiation by ages 20 and 21.

Partner Switching among Initiates

The cumulative partner acquisitions that were described in Chapter 12 and shown graphically in Figures 12.1 and 12.2 included both first and later partners. Having analysed initiations in some detail, and having shown that early initiation is correlated with a high overall rate of partner change, it is useful now to calculate the age-specific post-initiation rates, separately. This allows a more precise representation of sexual behaviour within a simulation model. That is, it allows us to separate primary initiation from subsequent behaviour. To carry out this calculation, the total number of partners contributing to the overall rate was reduced by one, and the denominator of years of experience was reduced by those years which preceded initiation.

For example, Table 12.1 has shown that 15-19 year-old males acquired 69.8 new partners, first or later, per 100 years of experience. Between the 15th and 20th birthday, each 100 subjects had accumulated 500 experience-years and acquired 349 partners (i.e. 69.8 x 5). First partners accounted for 74.8 of the 349 total partners (see Table 12.5) leaving 274.2 *subsequent* partners. The basic computer tabulations showed that these subsequent partners were encountered within a period of 217.7 post-first-partner experience years. This gives a post-initiation acquisition rate of 125.9 per 100 years of experience. This is about five times the mean rate of initiation which had preceded it.

In subsequent age groups, where most of the new encounters were among the initiated, the post-first-partner rates became closer to the values already calculated for total experience (Table 12.1). For example, in the age-band 20-24, the rate per 100 post-first-partner years declined from 125.9 to 59.1, little more than the *overall* partner-acquisition rate of 57.5. At later ages still this convergence was almost complete. For females aged 15-19 (lower panel of Table 12.1) the rate of acquisition of new partners after the first partner was 53.4 per 100 years of post-first-partner experience: about twice the preceding rate of initiation. In later age-bands it too corresponded closely with the overall partner acquisition rate.

The separate calculation of initiation rates and of post-initiation acquisition rates was carried out in the different social, demographic and educational groups. This showed that the greater parts of the gradients associated with these factors were related to the stage of acquiring subsequent rather than first partners. It conforms with the earlier finding that the social correlations with total partners were more powerful than those with first partners. Similar calculations showed the extent of the differences, in terms of their subsequent experiences, between those recording earlier and later first inter-course. The early starters shown in the first two panels of Table 12.3, with their high initiation rates, then continued with post-first-partner acquisition rates at about 200 per hundred years of experience: (2 new partners per person per annum). They then continued at rates not far short of this value for the 5 or 10 or more years for which they were followed.

Individual Variations

All partner acquisition rates have so far been expressed as mean values, but detailed tabulations showed that the variations within many of the social and demographic groups were as striking as the differences between them. There was a wide distribution around all of these means. Table 15.2 shows the distributions of numbers of subsequent sexual partners before the 20th birthday, among males and females who had first intercourse before their 16th birthday. Cohorts 5, 6 and 7 are shown separately, for males and for females. All the distributions showed extended tails at the high frequency end, especially among the males. About 39 percent of the early-starting males recorded 10 or more partners before they were 20: and 19 percent of the early-starting females. Ten percent of the males had recorded more than 25 partners by this age.

Table 15.2

Variation in numbers of partners between 15 and 19 years

Early starters (age 15) in Cohorts 5, 6, 7**

Number of subsequent partners	Males			Females		
	cohort 5	cohort 6	cohort 7*	cohort 5	cohort 6	cohort 7*
1	0	1	0	0	0	1
2	0	1	8	2	1	2
3	0	0	6	1	4	5
4	0	0	14	2	3	6
5	1	1	11	3	4	2
6	1	4	9	0	7	3
7	0	0	8	2	2	1
8	1	1	8	1	0	2
9	0	1	6	0	4	1
10	1	4	9	0	1	1
11	0	3	3	0	3	1
12	1	0	0	0	0	0
13	0	2	1	1	3	0
14	0	0	0	1	1	0
15	0	1	0	0	1	0
16-25	2	6	8	2	0	0
>25	2	8	2	0	0	0

*incomplete surveillance between 15 and 19 years

**Cohorts 5, 6, 7 = births in 1960-64, 1965-69, 1970-76.

These asymmetric distributions, with these wide variations of numbers of heterosexual partners, occurred in every social, demographic and educational class. They will have to be represented in some simplified manner when we come to enter them in our simulation model. It is sufficient for the time being to note that each of them could be represented roughly in the form of three separate groups. The first would comprise a central 50 percent with a mean value close to the overall mean; and with a lower 25 percent and upper 25 percent exhibiting half and double the average rates.

A further form of sharply differentiated individual variation in sexual behaviour was found among those engaged in marriages and in other cohabiting partnerships. So far as we could tell, the majority of such partners remain faithful, but a substantial proportion, 22 percent of the men and 18 percent of the women could be shown to have undertaken new sexual relationships during the course of the current one. A recent study from Norway (17) reports comparable figures, although measured in a different way; 15 percent of men and 9 percent of women living with a partner had engaged in 'extra-marital' sex during the previous three years.

Variation of Activity with Age

We have seen that initiation rates among the non-initiated rose with increasing age (Table 15.1). However, post-initiation rates of partner-acquisitions then rose immediately to their highest levels, and later declined with increasing age. Among males, the greatest absolute numbers of initiations were before the age of 16 and the greatest numbers of later partner acquisitions were occurring at age 17. Among the females in the sample, peak numbers of initiations were at ages 17 and 18, and the greatest numbers of later partner acquisitions began immediately after this age. The subsequent attenuation of later partner acquisitions continued for as long as the cohorts were followed but the rate of decline with increasing age was less in the later cohorts than in the early ones. The outcome was that the earlier cohorts were overtaken in terms of their cumulative numbers of partners by almost all of the later cohorts. This was illustrated in Figures 12.1 and 12.2.

Although the scale of the changes increased in successive cohorts, the general forms of the curves of partner acquisition were similar. The successive curves can be represented conveniently by declaring a 'peak' value which increases from one cohort to the next: and modifying this peak value at different ages in the terms of a Weibull distribution. The Weibull curve, as used here, is illustrated in Figure 15.1 and is represented algebraically as

$$r = t^c \exp (1\text{-}t^c)$$

where

      r = the relative annual rate of partner acquisition
      t is age, in the units described below
      c is a skew factor, which operates through distorting the age-scale

The unit of age is the interval between an initiating age (e.g. 15th birthday: corresponding with $t = 0$) and a peak age (e.g. 18th birthday: corresponding with $t = 1.0$). The unit in this example is 3 years. When $t = 0$ (e.g. 15th birthday) then $r = 0.0$. At the peak age, when $t = 1.0$ (e.g. 18th birthday) then $r = 1.0$. Thereafter, r declines towards 0.0.

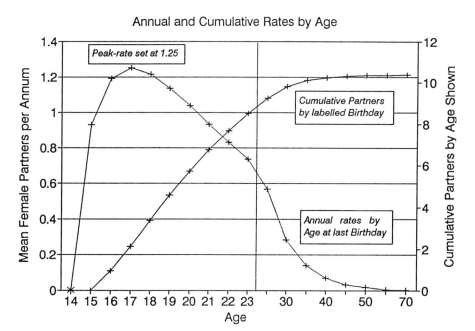

Figure 15.1

Weibull Model of Male Sexual Partnering

Annual and Cumulative Rates by Age

The calculated value 'r' is used to adjust the peak rate so as to calculate rates at other ages. The skew factor, c, adjusts the shape of the curve, raising it or lowering it everywhere except for its two fixed points, t=0 and t=1.0.

In addition to demonstrating this primary Weibull curve, Figure 15.1 also shows a cumulative curve analogous with those shown in Figures 12.1 and 12.2. The choice of parameters – the initiating age, the peak age and the skew parameter – for use in the model, is discussed later.

Male/Female Imbalance

We have seen that the males recorded higher rates of partner acquisition than did the females. This was consistent in all cohorts, at all ages, within each of the social, demographic and educational groups, at each age of first intercourse . . . and so on. It was present both for first partners and for later partners. We wondered at first whether the males had exaggerated or that the females were reticent, or both. However, our studies of internal consistencies of individual questionnaires showed no direct evidence of this. The men were less consistent than the women but this was probably secondary to their more complex sexual careers. Furthermore, the evidence on the durations of partnerships, both for males and for females, was consistent with their statements regarding the frequency of changing partners. All the evidence suggested that the inconsistencies were the inconsistencies of muddle rather than of deceit or of self deceit, and that another explanation for the gender-difference must be sought.

One alternative explanation, already presented, is an interaction between the different age preferences of males and females in seeking sexual partners and a rapid change in the activities of successive cohorts. It almost certainly accounts for part of the gender difference: but probably not all of it.

The remainder of the gender difference is probably due to different degrees of sampling bias. First, there were no self-admitted prostitutes among our sample of females and none with a history to suggest it. Much of the female deficit could be explained if we supposed, for example, that the true prevalence of prostitutes in the population was 3 to 4 per 1000 in the age group 15-50, and if they each accommodated 1000 different clients a year. However, the prostitute usage declared by the male respondents was much less than this and there was still a major gender difference within the sample when the admitted prostitute contacts were omitted from the calculation. If the sample was short of prostitutes, then it was also short of the clients of prostitutes.

A second form of sampling bias would arise if highly active females other than prostitutes had been selectively depleted from the working population from which our sample was drawn. The age preference distributions described in Chapter 13 (Table 13.2) suggest a mechanism. Few of the female respondents admitted to partnerships with the youngest males, particularly those of 17 years or less, although this was one of the most active age-bands for the male respondents. That is, the female sample is short of certain partnerships which were abundant among the records of the male sample: those in which both partners were less than 18 years of age. There is much parallel evidence to suggest that this depletion may be the result of pregnancy.

In 1989 in England and Wales the annual birth rate among women under 20 years of age was 32 per thousand. Registered pregnancy terminations (OPCS reports) increase the known pregnancy rate by a factor of 1.56, leading to a cumulative 248 pregnancies per 1000 women by the age of 20; or rather more if we allow for the lead time to deliveries occurring in the 21st year. In round numbers, and allowing for repeated pregnancies in some women, one quarter of all females resident in England and Wales in recent years have become pregnant by age 20.

Many of these young women are presumably absent from our working sample. They are among those with 'early-initiations' and with the highest rates of subsequent partner-acquisition and presumably the greatest pregnancy risks. The young fathers are also absent from the partnering-records of our female respondents (see Table 13.2). These young men are probably not capable of providing either economic support or a realistic prospect of marriage, and many of the pregnancies in the missing women are 'illegitimate'. In England and Wales in 1989, 78 percent of births to women under 20 were 'illegitimate'. The women absent from our sample, many with neither domestic nor independent financial support, are either unemployed and receiving benefits and engaged in their own domestic work, or are engaged in low paid work in those labour-intensive industries which we ourselves found difficult to access. The recent national increases in early pregnancies and in illegitimate births are presumably related to the accelerating behaviour changes noted in our own recent cohorts, and it seems likely that a major part of the gender imbalance in the sample may have occurred through this form of negative selection. That is, the gender imbalance represents a selective shortage of partners among the females, rather than a selective excess among the males.

From this it follows that our best estimates of rates of partner switching, in both sexes, are to be obtained from the rates represented in Figure 12.1. That is, the 1945-49 male cohort will probably terminate their sexual careers with a mean number of about 8 female partners; and the next two cohorts with about 9 or 10. The 1960-64 and later cohorts are heading for totals which we cannot yet measure: but probably 12 to 15 partners. For the females, we must suppose that the same figures will be reached about one quinquennial cohort later.

These estimates are rather greater than the incomplete partner-tallies reported in 1981 in a study of husbands of women with cervical pathologies, and controls (13). The ages of the husbands were not supplied, but given the fact of cervical carcinoma in the wives, which occurs most frequently at greater ages, they probably correspond behaviourly with the earlier cohorts of our own study: or perhaps earlier cohorts still. An investigation of the numbers of sexual partners among women attending a Family Planning Clinic at ages 25-49 also reported results corresponding with our own early cohorts. Social class and educational correlations similar to the ones we ourselves demonstrated in men, were also evident; and another report from the same group demonstrated the same false inversion of cumulative numbers of partners, with increasing current age, (see Fig. 9.2) as we have demonstrated in our own cross-sectional sample (12,14,15).

Risk Variations

Different partnerships which in superficial terms appear similar – same social class, same ages, same cohorts, same starting ages etc. – may differ widely in the risk of transmitting an infection present in one of the pair. The most obvious factors enhancing or ameliorating the risk of transmission are the frequency of sexual intercourse, the use of heterosexual anal intercourse, and the use or non-use of condoms.

Our measured intercourse frequencies were similar to values reported by Kinsey (18) where the mean frequency of intercourse among married persons was about 20 times per month; and among singles, about 6 times per month. The *inverse* relationship that we have shown between the frequency of intercourse and the frequency of partner change surprised us. Although the reasons behind it can be surmised, we have not encountered any similar observation in the scientific literature.

The usage of condoms over the greater part of the study period corresponded with findings reported in other studies. For example, a recent U.K. household survey of 5,000 men and women aged 16-55 (in 1990) reported 29 percent usage by males and 20 percent usage by females within the last 3 months. Greater condom use in casual partnerships compared with more durable partnerships, has also been noted before. However, the major increase of usage in the very latest cohorts observed in our sample exceeded the proportions noted in these and in other reports and is potentially of great importance (19,20,21,22).

We have found one recent British study reporting the frequency of heterosexual anal intercourse. Although this was not strictly comparable with our own, it elicited an admission of heterosexual anal intercourse in 14 percent of 20-year-olds (23). Unfortunately, these data were collected through a postal questionnaire with a response rate of only 37 percent. We have found nothing at all in the recent literature from this country to compare with our findings on the frequency of overlapping heterosexual partnerships.

Homosexual Behaviour

Among the sexually initiated men, there were 74 (6.9 percent) who reported homosexual or bi-sexual behaviour. This is similar to reports in other investigations from Kinsey onwards (18,24,25,26,27,28,29,30,31). However, there does not appear to be any recent well-founded estimate for this country as a whole, or any precise evaluation of the manner in which it varies in the different regions.

Our own questionnaire focussed particularly on the question of homosexual anal intercourse, the major risk factor of HIV transmission. Anal intercourse was recorded by only 44 (59 percent) of the 74 homosexual men: amounting to 4.1 percent of all sexually initiated men. Most of them (70 percent – 31) said that they had practised anal homosexual intercourse with fewer than 3 different partners: only 3 men reported more than 10 partners: and none reported more than 25. If these reports are to be believed, the highly promiscuous sexual behaviour described elsewhere, involving tens or hundreds of partners per year, and at the centre of the transmission pattern for HIV, was absent from this group. Our special pilot study of men sampled in various gay venues had shown higher partner rates, 20 percent of this group reporting more than 50 partners.

It is possible, that our sampling method had excluded many men engaged in these levels of homosexual behaviour. The only safe conclusion is that this survey gives insufficient material to estimate the prevalence of promiscuous homosexual behaviour in the population at large, or the proportion of bi-sexuals, or the extent of the sexual contacts between the bi-sexuals and heterosexual women.

We enquired about the use of homosexual male prostitutes. Only 2 of the men in the sample reported such usage.

Female Prostitution

None of the women in the sample volunteered that they were or had been prostitutes (although we did not specifically ask) and none of them reported numbers of partners sufficient to suggest that they might have been. Our evidence on the prevalence of prostitution, and the numbers of clients catered for, must come almost entirely from other sources.

There are serious difficulties in estimating the prevalences of persons in all 'hidden' classes – especially prostitutes and drug users (32,33) – but local studies among prostitutes have estimated that Birmingham, with its total population of 1.1 million persons, has approximately 1,000 prostitutes at any one time (34,35). Among approximately 250,000 Birmingham women in the age-band 15-50 years, this represents a prevalence of about 4 per 1,000. Less than half of these women operate entirely as 'street prostitutes' and the remainder operate through telephone contacts, saunas, escort agencies and clubs, hotels and other 'indoor' contacts: or through combinations of these methods and street soliciting.

Not all of them are working all of the time and they also accommodate clients from outside the City. In addition, more than half of them also worked, or had worked outside Birmingham. The currently-active prevalence relative to Birmingham male clients was therefore probably less than the simple estimate of prevalence might suggest: possibly 2.0 per 1,000 women. The numbers of clients accommodated by each female prostitute is likewise difficult to estimate. Street prostitutes in Birmingham reported widely varying numbers but the mean amounted to 22 clients per week: about 1100 per year. They reported condom usage in 91 percent of instances of vaginal intercourse.

We could not reconcile these values with the low usages reported by our respondents, and this may represent bias in our sample. Alternatively, the mode of contacting the prostitutes in the above study may have selected the more active ones; or the prostitutes may have overstated their activities; or their services may have been spread over clients from an even wider region than was thought. This created problems in setting parameters for our model. We describe this process later.

Conclusions

The pattern of sexual behaviour in this country, as judged by this West Midlands sample, is extremely variable. There are wide differences between social and demographic groups and equally wide differences within them, and patterns of partner-acquisition, condom usage, and early pregnancy are changing very rapidly indeed. Survey data obtained some time ago, or from other countries, can contribute little to an understanding of the current situation; and even recent data require extrapolation if they are to be used for predicting the spread of infection. Some of the social and demographic variations must strongly affect the structure of any samples extracted from the working population, and this was probably the major source of the gender differences in the reported sexual behaviour patterns. These selective processes, and the consequent bias, operated more severely upon the females than upon the males; but even for the males, the sample distributions suggest that rates of partner acquisition in the population as a whole must be greater than those derived from this investigation.

References

1. Knox E.G. (1986) 'A Transmission model for AIDS'. *Eur. J. Epidem.* **2**: 165-177.

2. Knox E.G. (1988) 'Modelling the AIDS Epidemic'. In: *Statistical Analysis and Mathematical Modelling of AIDS.* pp. 106-111. New York 1988.

3. Knox E.G. (1984) 'Epidemic Cancer of the Cervix'. In: *Hormones and sexual factors in human cancer aetiology.* Eds. J.P. Wolff and J.S. Scott.

4. Knox E.G. and Shannon H. (1988) 'Cancer of the cervix and the papilloma viruses'. *Eur. J. Epid.* **1**: 83-92.

5. Heisterkamp S.H., De Haan B.J., Jager J.C., Van Druten J.A.M. and Hendriks J.C.M. (1992) 'Short and medium term Projections of the AIDS/HIV Epidemic by a dynamic model with an application to the risk group of homo/bisexual men in Amsterdam'. *Statistics in Medicine* **11**: 1425-1441.

6. Anderson R.M. (1988) 'The Epidemiology of HIV Infection: Variable Incubation Plus Infectious Periods and Heterogeneity in Sexual Activity'. *J.R. Statist. Soc.* **151**: 66-93.

7. Jacquez J.A., Simon C.P., Koopman J., Sattenspiel L. and Perry T. (1988) 'Modeling and Analysing HIV Transmission: The Effect of Contact Patterns'. *Mathematical Biosciences* **92**: 119-199.

8. Grant R.M., Wiley J.A. and Winkelstein W. (1987) 'Infectivity of the human immunodeficiency virus: estimates from a prospective study of homosexual men'. *J. Infect. Dis.* **156**: 189-193.

9. Rolnick S.J., Gross C.R., Garrard J. and Gibson R.W. (1989) 'A Comparison of Response Rate, Data Quality and Cost in the Collection of Data on Sexual History and Personal Behaviours'. *Amer. J. Epidem.* **129**: 1052-1060.

10. MacArthur C., Lewis M., Knox E.G. and Crawford J.S. (1990) 'Epidural anaesthesia and long-term backache after childbirth'. *Brit. Med. J.* **301**: 9-12.

11. Central Statistical Office (1992) *Social Trends* **22,** HMSO.

12. Harris R.W.C., Brinton L.A., Cowdell R.H., Skegg D.C.G., Smith P.G., Vessey M.P. and Doll R. (1980) 'Characteristics of women with Dysplasia or Carcinoma in situ of the Cervix Uteri'. *Br. J. Cancer* **42**: 359-369.

13. Buckley J.D., Harris R.W.C., Doll R., Vessey M.P. and Williams P.T. (1981) 'Case-control study of the husbands of women with dysplasia or carcinoma of the cervix uteri'. *Lancet ii.* 1010-1015.

14. Brown S., Vessey M. and Harris R. (1984) 'Social class, sexual habits and cancer of the cervix'. *Community Medicine* **6**: 281-286.

15. Mant D., Vessey M. and Loudon N. (1988) 'Social class differences in sexual behaviour and cervical cancer'. *Community Medicine* **1**: 52-56.

16. La Vecchia C., Francheschi S., Decarli A., Fasoli M., Gentile A., Parazzine F., Regallo M. (1986) Sexual Factors, Venereal Diseases and the Risk of Intraepithelial and Invasive Cervical Neoplasia. *Cancer* **58**: 935-941.

17. Stigum H., Gronnesby J.K., Magnus P., Sundet J.M. and Bakketeig L.S. (1991) 'The Potential for spread of HIV in the Heterosexual Population in Norway: A Model Study'. *Statistics in Medicine* **10**: 1003-1023.

18. Kinsey A.C., Pomeroy W.B., Martom C.E. *Sexual Behaviour in the Human Male.* Philadelphia. 1948.

19. Robertson B.J., McQueen D.V. and Nisbet L. (1992) 'AIDS-related behaviours provisional data from the RUHBC CATI Survey. *Research Unit in Health and Behavioural Change,* **30**: University of Edinburgh.

20. Sundet J.M., Magnus P., Kvalem I.L., Gronnesby J.K. and Bakketeig L.S. (1989) 'Numbers of sexual partners and use of condoms in the heterosexual population of Norway – relevance to HIV-infection'. *Health Policy* **13**: 159-167.

21. L.R.C. Products Ltd. *The Durex Report* (1991).

22. Consumer Association. Which? (April 1989) *Time for some more condom sense.* 18-23.

23. Breakwell G.M. and Fife-Schaw C.R. (1991) 'Heterosexual anal intercourse and the risk of AIDS and HIV for 16-20 year-olds'. *Health Education Journal* **50:** 166-169.

24. Druten van J.A.M., Boo de Th., Reintjes A.G.M., Jager J.C., Heisterkamp S.H., Coutinho R.A., Bos J.M. and Ruitenberg E.J. 'Reconstruction and prediction of spread of HIV infection in populations of homosexual men'. In: *Statistical Analysis and Mathematical Modelling of AIDS.* Eds. J.C. Jager and E.J. Ruitenberg. Oxford University Press 1988.

25. Heisterkamp S.H., De Haan B.J., Jager J.C., Van Druten J.A.M. and Hendriks J.C.M. (1992) 'Short and medium term Projections of the AIDS/HIV Epidemic by a dynamic model with an application to the risk group of Homo/Bisexual men in Amsterdam'. *Statistics in Medicine* **11**: 1425-1441.

26. Fitzpatrick R., Boulton M., Hart G., Dawson J. and McLean J. (1989) 'High risk sexual behaviour and condom use in a sample of homosexual and bisexual men'. *Health Trends* **21**: 76-79.

27. McEvoy M. (1987) 'Homosexual activity data in the United Kingdom'. In: *Future Trends in AIDS*. A Seminar to discuss the prediction of the AIDS Epidemic. HMSO. London.

28. McManus T.K. and McEvoy M.B. (1987) 'Some aspects of male homosexual behaviour in the UK'. *Brit. J. Sexual Medicine*. **14** 110-118

29. Ebbesen P., Melbye M. and Biggar R.J. (1984) 'Sex Habits, recent disease, and drug use in two groups of Danish male homosexuals'. *Archives of Sexual Behaviour*. **13** 291-300.

30. Valdiserri R.O., Lyter D.W., Leviton L.C., Callahan C.M., Kingsley L.A. and Rinaldo C.R. (1989) 'AIDS prevention in homosexual and bisexual men: results of a randomized trial evaluating two risk reduction interventions'. *Current Science Ltd.* **3**: 21-26.

31. Golombok S., Sketchley J. and Rust J. (1989) 'Condom use among homosexual men'. *AIDS Care*. **1**: 27-33.

32. Bloor M., McKeganey N. and Barnard M. (1990) 'An ethnographic study of HIV-related risk practices among Glasgow rent boys and their clients: report of a pilot study'. *AIDS Care* **2**: 17-24.

33. McKeganey N., Barnard M. and Bloor M. (1990) 'A comparison of HIV-related risk behaviour and risk reduction between female street working prostitutes and male rent boys in Glasgow' *Sociology of Health and Illness* **12**: 274-292.

34. Kinnell H. (1990) 'Prostitutes and their clients in Birmingham: Action Research to Measure and Reduce Risks of HIV'. *Royal Society of Medicine* **19**: 1-3.

35. Kinnell H. (1990) *Personal Communication*.

PART THREE

Dynamics of Transmission

Chapter 16 – An outline of the model

The computer simulator described here is a compartmental model. In this respect it resembles all previous HIV transmission models described in Part I of this book. The compartments hold numbers of individuals of different genders, different ages, different sexual preferences, different levels of sexual activity and different HIV-infective or susceptible states. Annual transfers between the compartments are determined first by demographic data derived mainly from birth/death/marriage/divorce registrations, describing processes in the population which the model represents. Further inter-compartmental transfers are then determined through 'natural history' movements from one HIV-state to another; and in response to the 'mass action' laws of infective transmission.

By 'mass action' we mean that within any socially-localised part of the population, the numbers of new infections occurring in each year are proportional to a) the numbers of infective persons present at the beginning of the year, b) the numbers of susceptibles with whom they come in contact, c) the durations of their relationships, and d) the annual rate of infectious transfer between partners, across the durations of their associations. Rates of partner change and the durations of partnerships are derived from the survey results already reported. Estimates of transmission risks have to be derived from observations on other populations, and through 'fitting' epidemic predictions to epidemic observations in our own.

This model is characterised chiefly by the complexity of its compartmentalisation. It is this which differentiates it from most other models, although there are some which approach its complexity (1,2). This requirement was imposed by the results of the population analysis already described, and the extreme variations of sexual styles and of partner change frequencies in different age groups, in different social, ethnic and educational groups, and in different birth cohorts: and indeed *within* each of these groups as well.

The model operates in discrete annual steps and in single annual age groups. This pattern was adopted in order to achieve a reasonable compromise between the need for computing power and storage space on the one hand, and the necessities for mimicking a rather slow epidemic process, on the other. This, together with careful design of data structures, and some compression of low-frequency classes, enabled implementation on a powerful Personal Computer rather than a mainframe or a supercomputer. The flexible development and transferability which this choice brings has been noted by other workers following similar paths (1, 2, 3). The main characteristics of the model are presented below in outline form, while details of the compartmental structure and a technical description of the infective transmission function, within the structure, are described in Appendix A16.

The inputs to the model consist of a range of demographic and biological parameters. They are entered through an interactive menu system.

The Structure of the Model: Setting up

At birth, the numbers of males and of females are each represented as '1.0': from which position they are dispersed, year by year, to different civil states, different behavioural levels and styles, and different HIV states. The initial population is structured by running the demographic processes across all the age bands, executing comulative demographic transfers at each step.

At later stages, representing successive calendar-years of the epidemic process, the demographic transfers are repeated, while at the same time a further level of disaggregation is executed. Within each age group, each gender, each behavioural style, and each class of partner-change frequency, the model-population is distributed as necessary according to HIV status. This goes beyond a simple infective/susceptible dichotomy. In addition to the 'susceptible' state, the taxonomy includes three successive stages of pre-AIDS HIV infection, as well as AIDS itself. Each stage has its own duration, rate of progression and infectivity level. A sixth class, 'immune', was included to permit simulation experiments with vaccines.

At the setting up stage, the HIV infection process is inhibited, but once the population has been established the epidemic is initiated by prescribing an initial 'seeding'. This involves transfers from susceptibles to infecteds at particular ages and in nominated sub-classes of the population – for example homosexuals, prostitutes and the most promiscuous heterosexual classes. The seedings are prescribed through the menu-driven input system. As the simulated epidemic proceeds, and as infected persons accumulate, the natural history of the infection is executed by transferring individuals (i.e. decimal fractions of groups) from one HIV class to the next; and finally to 'dead from AIDS'. This class is accumulated separately from 'dead from other causes', which provides a competitive form of exit from the population.

All transfer rules are deterministic. Random-number-based processes are not used.

Demographic Structure of the Population

The initial age structure of the population is constructed from the male and female L_x columns of the life table for the population to be mimicked. The population is held in separate single-year age groups labelled according to age at last birthday – 0 to 87 – at which latter age all remaining survivors are terminated. At the end of each annual cycle, each age group is 'aged' by one year and simultaneously decremented according to the D_x column of the life table. Newborns are introduced to refill the 0-year gap thus created. Initially, the newborns are all susceptible but, as the epidemic proceeds, a proportion become infected from their HIV-positive mothers. From 15 years of age onwards, surviving males and females are 'married' and 'divorced' according to the primary marriage rates, divorce rates and secondary marriage rates of the simulated population. All these demographic data are held in an accessory input file, which can be edited to suit the population which is to be mimicked. There is provision for the entry of two marriage advantage/disadvantage parameters. One modifies the celibate marriage rate compared with that among the sexually active – the latter being taken as 'standard'. The other modifies marriage rates among homosexuals and bi-sexuals, relative to active heterosexuals.

In real populations, the L_x distribution differs from the current age profile of the population. This is unlikely to perturb the operation of the model in any important respect but it would be a simple matter to modify the age-specific printed results in terms of the true profile, if this were desired.

The different behaviour patterns of married and unmarried men and women, and (possibly) differing transmission risks within and outside marriage, required separate identification and treatment of married pairs. In order to do this, the model transfers marrying men into the 'female' half of the population table, in association with their wives. 'Marrying women' are transformed into 'married couples', and the men disappear from the male half of the table. Death of either partner of a marriage results in a re-dispersal of the survivor to an uncoupled state in the appropriate half of the population, while divorce or separation results in dispersal of both partners. Surviving females remain within their 'married' age group, while separated men are shifted upwards in accordance with the mean age difference between husbands and wives, returning them to the age group to which they belong.

Partner-change frequencies of single persons are defined at three activity levels (see p 175–6) and extra-marital contacts of unfaithful married men and of unfaithful married women are treated as for the unmarried. Married pairs are classified to nine combinations of their extramarital activity levels, derived from three assigned to the husbands and three assigned to the wives. The nine frequencies are the products of the individual (3x3) frequencies, modified through a behavioural correlation parameter. All values are entered through the 'menu system'.

The contact and transmission rules between married couples are different from those relating to singles. Partly to compensate for the extended behavioural classification of married couples, the three pre-AIDS HIV-states in marrieds are compressed to a single state with a composite duration and infectivity. The six basic infectivity states are thus reduced to four: and the potential 36 husband/wife combinations, to just 16.

It would be possible within this format to redefine a proportion of the singles contacts as 'effectively married'. This would require simply an increase in the state of marriage rates, and possibly the divorce rates as well. However, this device was not used in any of the simulations described later.

Behavioural Stratification

The behavioural classification of persons in different marital states, and the rates at which they change their partners, are entered to the program through a series of menus. The menu texts, associated with default values, are held in accessory files which are called down in sequence. Each menu invites the user to replace the given values with those of his/her choice. Replacement values are used only for the particular run of the model and are not copied back to the accessory files. However, these files can be edited external to the program itself, if particular default values are to be 'immortalised'. The menu-displays in the accessory files are written in English, but could be translated to other languages.

Menus specifying sexual behaviour list the proportions of persons adopting different sexual styles and the proportions adopting one of three different levels of partner-change frequency within each of these styles (see p 175–6). The proportions adopting the different sexual styles and levels are specified separately for married, single and divorced/widowed men and women. Further menus attach absolute values of annual partner-change frequencies to all these classes. Age-specific rates of sexual initiation among celibates of both sexes are also entered; likewise, the frequency of usage and the efficacy of condoms in different behavioural classes. The term 'efficacy' is construed here as a joint measure of a) the reliability of the condoms themselves, and b) the regularity of use and the technical proficiency of usage, among 'users'.

Rates of partner change among sexually active men and women are modified for each birth cohort, and continually within the cohort according to age. The basic cohort modifiers, and the parameters for a Weibull age-modification (specified later) are entered by menu. The age preferences of partners according to the age and gender of the seeker, and proportions of faithful husbands and faithful wives are entered in a similar manner.

The behaviour structure of the model-population is non-orthogonal. That is, it has a branched format with different levels of elaboration in different branches. For example, active single females are distributed to two sexual styles ('selective' and 'prostitute') and active males to seven separate styles; and each style of each gender is distributed to three levels of partner-change activity. Divorced/widowed males and females are each accommodated in a single (presumed heterosexual) style: again with three activity levels. Married couples are distributed according to the seven corresponding sexual styles of unfaithful husbands: but nine different combinations of activity level, as described. Altogether, each annual age-band is elaborated to 166 behavioural/demographic classes: the whole then repeated six-fold for the different infectivity states. The detailed specification of this structure is set out in Appendix A16.

Balancing the Activities

The frequencies of the styles and levels, and the corresponding partner-acquisition rates, are declared in an arbitrary manner in the sense that each specification is made without necessary reference to the others with which it interacts. In addition, activity levels are modified as the epidemic evolves and different behavioural classes are depleted or augmented at different and changing rates. In practical terms, the 'seeking' and the available 'reciprocating' elements of sexual behaviour, across the population, never match each other exactly. This technical problem was encountered in our previous equilibrium model (see Part I of this book) and the problem is even more complex in a dynamic model where the population structure is continually modified, and the internal processes continually changed.

This problem is handled through a preliminary scan of the entire population from age-0 to age-87, at each annual cycle, prior to the execution of any demographic movements, sexual contacts, infections and natural-history shifts. This scan sums the frequencies of the various styles of activity sought, on the basis of the entered behavioural characteristics, modified by age and by cohort, and the current frequencies of the various 'seeker' classes. These sums identify the imbalances between the female-seeking activities of heterosexual and bisexual single and married men: the mixed heterosexual and bisexual male-seeking activities of the women: and the anal penetrative and receptive-seeking activities of single-preference and mixed-preference homosexuals and bisexuals. On the basis of these identified imbalances, a set of activity-modifiers is calculated, and used during the 'business' scan to bring activities into a proper balance. In effect, the seeking behaviours entered through the menus are treated as bargaining positions, and the program computes the best accommodation of conflicting desires.

The preliminary 'counting' scan also calculates the HIV-stage distribution associated with each of the four basic seeking activities; namely, female-seeking by men, male-seeking by females, penetrative homosexual-seeking, and receptive homosexual-seeking. The results are stored with the age-group record and used later to represent reciprocating availabilities among partners sought and taken up by seekers from other age groups. The counting scan also calculates and stores a compounded transfer risk, based jointly on the HIV stage-distribution, the relative risks associated with each of these stages, and the absolute transfer risks associated with particular seeking/reciprocating combinations.

The 'mass-action' Infection Process

The mass-action process determines the numbers of infections occurring during each year in each age group in all the separate classes. It is executed at each annual cycle in 88 separate steps, as the entire age-distributed population is scanned. Transfers from 'susceptible' to 'infected' depend on three separate parameters namely the rate of new partner acquisition within the class (*a*), the prevalence of infectives among the partners of susceptibles (*b*), and the compounded transfer risk per unit time, as described above (*c*). Each class, each sexual style, each activity level in the singles, and each combination of husband/wife activity levels among married couples, is processed in turn. The process focuses upon the susceptibles, negotiating their partner types and ages according to the rules, and adjusting each of the transfer-determining parameters to the local situation, at each step. The component activities of susceptibles with mixed preferences are examined separately.

Rates of partner-change (parameter *a*) are modified at each age-step of each annual cycle according to the age-dependent Weibull function, and also according to birth cohort. The proportion of infectives among their partners (parameter *b*) is based upon counting the HIV stage-distributions stored in the age groups and behaviour-types from which the partners are selected, and weighting them appropriately. The partners' age groups themselves are identified through a regression equation entered by the menu system. 'Risk on contact' (parameter *c*) is recalculated for each style of susceptible (female-seeking by men, male-seeking by females, penetrative homosexual-seeking, receptive homosexual-seeking), each with its specific predeclared risk, and upon the current distribution of the different HIV states among available and appropriate partners.

Because prostitutes incur special risks deriving from the high risk sexual behaviours of their clients, and the use of drugs both by clients and the prostitutes themselves, a menu facility was provided whereby infectivity *to* prostitutes *from* clients could be augmented. The default value is set at 3.0.

The risk of transfer from susceptible to infected during the course of a year depends jointly upon these three parameters, a, b and c, and the transfer function is calculated as . . .

$$1-[1-b(1-e^{-c/(a+1)})]^{(a+1)}$$

The derivation of this basic expression is demonstrated in Part 2 of Appendix A16 and is validated through comparison with alternative formats, in Parts 3 and 4. This formula takes account of the risk of acquiring an infection from the partner current at the beginning of a year, as well as from new partners. Sexual initiation and marriage are not themselves construed as risks, but risk exposure begins immediately afterwards.

The question arose whether those with high rates of partner change would also have high rates of sexual contact within their partnerships – a recurring 'honeymoon period'; and whether this would require an additional adjustment to the transmission formula. In the event, the supposition was not born out by the facts, and the adjustment was not necessary. However, it also seemed likely that individuals with high rates of partner change might tend to seek partners of the same type and therefore with high prevalences of infective states. That is, there would be a local correlation between b and a. The use of a single value of b for different levels of a would not then suffice. We return to this issue later.

Natural History

The natural history sequence of the program is executed before the mass action infection sequence. If it were otherwise, then new infections would be 'moved on' instantly to the next HIV-stage without having had a chance to infect others. The natural history sequence is itself managed in reverse order, for similar reasons. Thus, a proportion of the AIDS cases dies and the residual AIDS cases are then augmented by transfers from the third stage of HIV infection. The third stage is then augmented by transfers from Stage 2; and Stage 2 by transfers from Stage 1. Rates of transfer from one stage to the next are customarily determined as the reciprocals of the mean durations of the donor stages. If a stage lasts five years, then the annual rate of transfer from that stage to the next one is taken to be 0.2. In practice, however, we encountered a complication which we had not foreseen, and which has important consequences.

In the early years of exponential growth, there are relatively few subjects in the advanced stages of the disease and relatively more in the early stages. The same applies to the individual years of a particular stage, so that the proportion eligible for transfer from one stage to the next is much less than the reciprocal of the mean duration of the stage. The use of unmodified reciprocals within a model is appropriate only to the eventual 'steady state'.

The model natural history process was adapted to take account of the phenomenon. It maintains a running record of the wedge shaped natural history distribution from the stage of 'seeding', onwards. This allows a correct determination of the proportions currently in the final years of each stage, and therefore eligible for transfer to the next.

The asymmetric stage-distribution during a period of rapid increase can interact with overall infectivity. For example, if the early stages are relatively infectious, then the mean infectivity is greater when the disease is increasing rapidly, than when it has attained a steady state. It is not clear how far this has been recognized, or taken into account in analyses of current data. It is certain, however, that the level of infectiousness in the earliest years of the natural history must play the dominant role in determining the rate of growth of the epidemic. Anderson (4) has commented briefly and accurately on this issue, although we were not aware of this until later. If the early stages are indeed relatively infectious, so that rapid growth increases infectiousness, while a level prevalence results in a decline, then we should expect the system to generate oscillations.

There are many expositions in the scientific literature of the effects of individual variations of natural history progressions. That is, the early years of the AIDS epidemic are dominated by individuals with relatively short natural histories, and this contributes to an accelerated evolution in the early years of the epidemic. But this point is entirely separate from that outlined above.

Extraction of Results

At each age-cycle the numbers in different classes and in different age-group/sexes were accumulated, and a similarly categorised total of person years at risk was assembled for different ages.

Each infective transfer from susceptibles to Stage-1 HIV infection, was monitored, accumulated, and assembled in the same format as the population denominators. The same was done for transfers from Stage-3 HIV to AIDS, from AIDS to dead from AIDS, for the current prevalence of HIV infection, and for the current prevalence of AIDS. At the end of each calendar year, when every age has been processed, the calculated rates per 100,000 population within each age, gender and behaviour group, are printed out directly: or temporarily to a disk file. Several different formats are used, including a disk file presentation in the 'comma format' used by spread-sheets. This permits ready transfer of results for use by spread-sheet graphic facilities.

APPENDIX A16

1. The Structure of the Population

The different demographic and behavioural types are held within a non-orthogonal branched structure with different levels of elaboration in the different branches. Active single females are distributed to two sexual styles ('selective' and 'prostitute') and active males to seven separate styles; and each style of each sex is distributed to three levels of activity. Divorced/widowed males and females are each accommodated in a single (presumed heterosexual) style: again with three activity levels. Married couples are distributed according to the seven corresponding sexual styles of unfaithful husbands: but nine joint extra-marital activity levels, representing three each for unfaithful husbands and unfaithful wives.

The unmarrieds are classified to one of six HIV-states. They include 1) susceptible, 2),3),4) successive stages of pre-clinical HIV disease, 5) AIDS, and 6) vaccine-immune. States 2 to 5 have separately designated durations and infectivities. Married men and married women are classified only to four states, the three pre-clinical stages having been compressed to a single state with a composite duration and a composite infectivity.

The population structure is accommodated in a programming entity known as a 'record'. Just as an 'array' is an assembly of elements of a similar type: so a 'record' is an assembly of elements of different types. It is this which allows different levels of elaboration in different branches. This in turn allowed selective compression and concatenation of classes and of interactions in less critical zones, with major economies in terms of storage and computer time. The simulation system was accommodated in a personal computer with additional storage space and 386/387 processors. Simulations were run at about two minutes per calendar year. The requirement for a 'record' structure led to the selection of a computer language capable of accommodating this format, and available on a micro-computer. The programme is written in PASCAL. The record structure representing the population is set out in Figure 16.1A.

2. The 'mass action' infection process

The risk of transfer from susceptible to infected depends jointly upon three parameters, a, b and c. Parameter-a is the rate of acquisition of new partners, after the first partner. Parameter-b is the prevalence of HIV-infectivity among partners. Parameter-c is the level of infectivity among infective partners, the estimate taking account of the type of sexual contact (heterosexual, homosexual) and the distribution of the infective partners

Figure 16.1A

```
Const                 { Structure-Determining Constants}
  C_male_style   =7;{ in order .. v,vp,vr,vpr,p,r,pr .....
                      sole style for active singles and
                      extramarital style for unfaithful husbands.}
  C_female_style=2;{ in order .. selective,prostitute.}
  C_HIV          =6;{ 6 Layers of T_Allstyle holding different HIV-States.
                      In singles: 1=suseptible(s);2,3,4=3 levels of HIV+(h);
                      5=AIDS(A);6=immune(i).   Dead-of-AIDS held separately.

                      In mpair1(male 1st):  1=ss;2=sh;3=sa;4=as;5=aa;6=ii;
                      In mpair2        :    1=hh;2=hs;3=si;4=is;5=ah;6=ha;
                      In DeadNAf       :    3=ih;4=iA;5=hi;6=Ai;
                      .. where h = H1+H2+H3  in singles; and full 6*6=36
                                              reduced to 4*4=16 in marrieds.}
  C_activity =  3;{ 3 levels, defined differently for different classes.}
  C_rec      = 192;{Elements in T_styleset. 166 compartments + 26 sums }
Type
  T_basic{4-byte}= single; {used for behaviour-type record .. T_styleset}
{*****************Range-setting section.***************************** }
  R_male_style   = 1..C_male_style;    {7}
  R_female_style = 1..C_female_style;  {2}
  R_activity     = 1..C_activity;      {3}
  R_HIV          = 1..C_HIV;           {6}
  R_26           = 1..26;                {26 subtotals at end of record}
{ ******************* Record-building section. ***********************}
  T_mstyle      = array[R_male_style]   of T_basic;
  T_fstyle      = array[R_female_style] of T_basic;
  T_levels      = array[R_activity]     of T_basic;          { 3 elements}
  T_levelM      = array[R_activity,R_activity] of T_basic; {9}
  T_singlesm    = array[R_male_style]   of T_levels;{ 7*3 = 21 elements}
  T_singlesf    = array[R_female_style] of T_levels;{ 2*3 =  6 elements}
  T_couples     = array[R_male_style]   of T_levelM;  {(7)*(3*3)=63}
  T_recd_tots   = array[R_26]           of T_basic;

  T_styleset    = Record {holds following 12 types}
  {no subscript} deadNAm:T_basic ;    {1:  1 element   dead,NotAIDS,male}
  {no subscript} deadNAf:T_basic ;    {2:  1 element   dead,NotAIDS, fem}
  {no    "     } celibm :T_basic;     {3:  1 element       uninitiated}
  {no    "     } celibf :T_basic;     {4:  1 element       uninitiated}
  { 1    "     } needle :T_levels;    {5:  3 elements              IVDU}
  { 1    "     } divorm :T_levels;    {6:  3 elements   divorced/widower}
  { 1    "     } divorf :T_levels;    {7:  3 elements   divorced/widow  }
  { 2    "     } acsfem :T_singlesf;  {8:  6 elements active single fem}
  { 2    "     } acsmal :T_singlesm;  {9: 21 elements active single mal}
  { 3+1  "     } mpair1 :T_couples;   {10: 63 elements     married pairs}
  { 3+1  "     } mpair2 :T_couples;   {11: 63 elements     married pairs}
  { 1    "     } totals :T_recd_tots; {12: 26 elements     summary-totals}
                 end;
  { Sum=192 of T_basic.  = 768 bytes in 4-byte 'singles' = 6 blocks*128
            alternatively 1152 bytes in 6-byte 'reals'  = 9 blocks*128}
  T_allstyle     = array [R_HIV] of T_styleset;   {6 HIV-layers of above}
                      { 6*192 of T_basic in T_Allstyle ....
                      = 36 or 54 128-blocks  for single or real.
                      = 4608 or 6912 bytes,  for single or real.
                  Assuming 27 * T_Allstyle in HEAP at one time, this requires
                          124416 bytes for single;        186628 bytes for real.
            89 FILE-RECORDS AT 4608 EACH  = 410126 bytes in RAM for single
                      or 6912 EACH  = 615168 bytes in RAM for real.  }
  T_Ptr_to_year = ^T_allstyle;{ points to 6-fold heap-block for 1 year.}
```

among the different HIV stages. Parameter 'c' is expressed per annum. The calculation of infective transfer takes account of the durations of the partnerships as well as the frequencies of change. The annual transfer function is derived as follows.

A group acquiring new partners at an annual rate of 'a', will on average be in contact with $(a+1)$ partners between the first day and the last day of each year. The mean duration of those contacts is $1/(a+1)$, if we assume that each one begins immediately after the termination of the previous one. This is not always true, some serial partnerships having gaps, and others having overlaps, but our data suggest that for our present purposes these alternatives can be regarded as cancelling out.

When a susceptible person is in contact with an infective person for $1/(a+1)$ years, the susceptible survives the exposure with a probability of

$$....e^{-c/(a+1)}$$

The complementary risk of being infected is $\quad ....1-e^{-c/(a+1)}$

If the partner of a susceptible is of unknown HIV status, selected from a population with an HIV-prevalence of b, the risk of being infected is

$$.....b(1-e^{-c/(a+1)})$$

and the survival probability is $\qquad .....1-b(1-e^{-c/(a+1)})$

Survival across $(a+1)$ separate contacts is $.....[1-b(1-e^{-c/(a+1)})]^{(a+1)}$

From this we calculate the risk of becoming infected from one or other of $(a+1)$ contacts as $\qquad .....1-[1-b(1-e^{-c/(a+1)})]^{(a+1)}$

This is the basic expression governing stepwise annual infectious transfer, within the model. Parameter 'b' must be in the range zero to 1.0 while parameters 'a' and 'c' can hold any non-negative value. Where a is small, approaching zero, and representing a partnership of indefinite length with no switching, the expression reduces to $b(1-e^{-c})$.

3. An alternative mass action function

The transfer function derived in the previous section uses a mean partner-switching rate, and takes no account of variation. In this section we disperse the numbers of new partner switches within the year according to the terms of a Poisson distribution. The separate terms are:-

New partners in year	Poisson term		Number-specific transfer function
0	e^{-a}	.	$b(1-e^{-c})$
1	$e^{-a}a$	.	$1-[1-b(1-e^{-c/2})]^2$
2	$e^{-a}a^2/2$	.	$1-[1-b(1-e^{-c/3})]^3$
3	$e^{-a}a^3/6$	.	$1-[1-b(1-e^{-c/4})]^4$
n	$e^{-a}a^n/n!$	.	$1-[1-b(1-e^{-c/(n+1)})]^{(n+1)}$

The sum of these terms was evaluated for a range of a, b and c, and the outcome compared with similar evaluations for the earlier non-distributed transfer function. The earlier format always exceeded the distributed format, usually by a factor between 1.005 and 1.02: no more than might have occurred through rounding errors, or the omission of higher Poisson terms. The Poisson expansion therefore offers no advantages over the unexpanded form.

There is no prior expectation that the distribution will be Poisson; indeed, the evidence of the survey is that the distribution will be wider, with a relative excess of low-n and high-n transfer terms. However, the differences between the expanded Poisson transfer terms were small, within the range of interest, and such as to minimise the effects of departures from a Poisson distribution.

4. The effects of discontinuities

Although the mean-based and the Poisson-expanded transfer functions relate to periods of exposure, and not partnerships, it seemed possible that the repeated use of this formula in successive years, with $(a+1)$ contacts each year, might in effect over-represent the long-term total of new partner acquisitions. A priori, the risk is ameliorated by the fact that a, as used here, is strictly the rate of *post-initiation* partner-acquisitions; also because the mean duration of all partnerships was short, less than 3 years. Nevertheless, we explored the possibility of error by re-calculating the results for extended time periods, greater than one year: and then comparing the results with the annual calculations (as above) repeated over the same number of separate years. The comparisons over a 3-year term are shown in Table A16.1. The differences were trivial, confirming that the transfer algorithm operates satisfactorily within this context, and that the annual stepwise discontinuity invokes no unacceptable errors.

5. Additional note

Over most of the parameter space, the use of a as index, instead of $(a+1)$, made little difference to the results. It also abolished the continuity problem, and therefore appears

Table A16.1

Ratios (Z)* between Annual Transfer Function Repeated over 3 years (Q) and Recalculated Value for a Continuous 3 years (S)**

a=0.2

		b	
c	0.01	0.02	0.10
0.02	1.010	1.010	1.009
0.05	1.026	1.026	1.023
0.07	1.036	1.036	1.033
0.10	1.052	1.051	1.047
0.15	1.067	1.066	1.061

a=0.5

		b	
c	0.01	0.02	0.10
0.02	1.005	1.005	1.005
0.05	1.013	1.013	1.012
0.07	1.018	1.018	1.017
0.10	1.026	1.026	1.024
0.15	1.034	1.034	1.031

a=1.0

		b	
c	0.01	0.02	0.10
0.02	1.002	1.002	1.002
0.05	1.006	1.006	1.006
0.07	1.009	1.009	1.008
0.10	1.012	1.012	1.011
0.15	1.016	1.016	1.014

*Z is calculated as follows

i) $P = 1-[1-(1-e^{-c/(a+1)})]^{(a+1)}$
$Q = 1-(1-P)^3$
ii) $S = 1-[1-(1-e^{-3c/(3a+1)})]^{(3a+1)}$
iii) $Z = Q/S$

**For a ten-year period, for both transfer functions, the proportional excesses are about three times those shown here. For example, 1.015 in place of 1.005. The only serious discrepancies between the two functions are for low a and high c, in combinations which do not occur in this context.

attractive. However, the transmission function then tends to zero as a tends to zero, instead of to $b(1-e^{-c})$. This option therefore fails to cater for groups of stable partnerships, including marriages, with very low rates of partner-switching, but in which one partner may already have been infected. This is an important group, and the need to represent it properly led us eventually to accept the $(a+1)$ index, despite its lack of generality and the small inaccuracies which it introduced.

Chapter 17 – Setting the Parameters of the Model

The model first executes a 'setting up' procedure to establish the initial population structure. It then runs in annual cycles for as long as is required. Both stages draw their demographic parameters from an ancillary data file and they draw their sexual behaviour parameters, natural history parameters and infectivity parameters through an interactive menu system. The menu texts and their default values are also held in ancillary files. This chapter describes the content of these data sources.

Demographic Parameters

The ancillary file DEMOGDAT.HIV is established and if necessary edited outside the operation of the program itself. It contains gender-specific mortality rates for England and Wales for 1987-89 together with rates of first marriages, divorce rates and rates of later marriages: all in 5-year age bands. The values used are shown in Table 17.1. The proportions of males and females in each marital state are calculated from these rates and are held within the program as decimal fractions of an initial unit value. Aging is handled at the end of each annual run by moving all values up by one year of age, and births are represented by inserting unit values for males and females at age-0. This renewal process does not use the absolute birth rates at different maternal ages but enters a constant number of births each year. It is designed to maintain a steady demographic structure. However, the maternal age-distribution of E&W births, also supplied in DEMOGDAT.HIV, combined with the current age-distribution of HIV positives among females in the model, determines the proportion of the new births which are at risk of HIV transfer from the mother.

These demographic parameters have been held constant throughout the simulations reported here. If a simulation is required for a country other than the UK, the source-file can be changed.

Sexual Initiation

Age-specific rates of sexual initiation among unmarried celibates are entered by menu. The default values, given in Table 17.2, were used unchanged for all the simulations reported. The values were based upon the survey results, although an adjustment was

Table 17.1

Demographic Data by Age Band

	Ages																	
	0-4	5-9	10-14	15-19	20-24	25-9	30-4	35-9	40-4	45-9	50-4	55-9	60-4	65-9	70-4	75-9	80-4	85-9
Deaths/100,000 p.a.																		
males	232	23	22	72	86	82	96	139	198	353	601	1070	1914	3156	5182	8048	12265	18100
females	178	16	16	31	32	36	55	90	140	230	370	650	1110	1780	2914	4670	7932	13148
First marriage/10,000 bachelors																		
males	–	–	–	47	547	904	751	405	212	122	75	25	(16)	(16)	(16)	(16)	(16)	(16)
females	–	–	–	188	916	1004	716	370	192	123	71	11	(6)	(6)	(6)	(6)	(6)	(6)
Re-marriage/10,000 divorced/widow(er)s																		
males	–	–	–	1018	1018	1333	1224	908	908	617	617	155	155	111	50	20	10	5
females	–	–	–	1391	1391	1402	1045	661	661	347	347	124	64	32	16	8	4	2
Divorces/10,000 married																		
males	–	–	–	70	26	316	261	208	164	124	68	68	16	9	5	3	2	1
females	–	–	–	102	284	290	230	182	140	101	48	48	12	8	4	2	1	1
Birth rates/10,000																		
women	–	–	–	301	927	1240	781	246	48	0								

Numbers living at different ages (0, 5, 10 . . .) are obtained by subtracting cumulative deaths from an original 100,000 born.
For example, at age 5, there are 100,000–232×5 male survivors

() Nominal values in parentheses

All rates are per annum

174

Table 17.2

Sexual Initiation Rates by Age

Model Parameters

Age at last birthday

	15-16	17-18	19-20	21-22	23-24	25+
Male	0.25	0.29	0.36	0.43	0.50	0.70
Female	0.20	0.26	0.31	0.36	0.36	0.36

These rates are simple proportions per annum per survivor. That is, 25 percent of 15 year-old males convert before age 16: another 25 percent of the remainder by age 17: and 29 percent of the remainder between 17 and 18: and again between 18 and 19. Marriages are drawn both from initiates and from celibates. Rates in celibates can be modified, relative to rates in initiates, using an advantage/disadvantage parameter. The default value is 1.0. Similarly, marriage rates among homosexual/bi-sexual males can be modified through the use of another parameter; again, this was set by default at 1.0.

made to allow for observed variations according to social and demographic character-istics, and the evident bias of the sample in these respects.

Marriages are executed both among the initiated and the non-initiated, the latter supplying an alternative form of initiation. An advantage/disadvantage parameter modifying the marriage rates of celibates relative to the initiated is available in the menu system but was held at unity in all the simulations reported. A second advantage/disadvantage parameter modifies the marriage risks of homosexuals and bi-sexuals relative to heterosexual males. The default value is also unity, but experimental variations are reported later.

Behavioural Styles and Activity-levels

The program allocates sexually active males, both single and married, to seven different 'sexual styles'. These are heterosexuals, three styles of bi-sexuals and three styles of homosexuals engaging in anal intercourse. These three styles are penetrative, receptive, and both. Separate menu entries determine the ratio of penetrative to receptive among those practising both; and the ratio of heterosexual to homosexual activities among the bi-sexuals. The default values were 1:1 in each case.

Single active females were allocated to one of two styles labelled as 'selective' and 'prostitute'. At the same time, the program allocates all sexually active singles, widowed/divorced and non-faithful marrieds to one of three levels of partner-changing activity. Level-1 is the least active, and Level-3 the most active. Married couples have nine different activity combinations, determined jointly by the separate distributions for the husbands and wives, and by a menu-entered 'correlation' parameter which links a high level in one with a high level in the other. This represents an assumption that men with high levels of extramarital activity tend to be married to women who also have high levels. The menus also invite entry of the proportion of husbands and wives who are 'faithful', and the activity-level classification operates only in relation to the 'non-faithful'. The default values for 'faithfulness' were 0.65, for both spouses. 'Faithful' means faithful this year: next year may be different for the individual, although the proportion remains constant.

The proportional values established for an initial set of experiments (described later) are set out in Table 17.3. The actual rates of partner change attached to each of the three activity levels are entered separately and are also described later.

Provision was initially made within the program for the entry of 'career-shift' parameters – rates of transfer between homosexual and heterosexual, or between prostitute and non-prostitute, for example. In the event, the available data proved inadequate for setting these parameters and the facility was abandoned. However, the program executes certain types of career-shift automatically. On marriage, the extra-marital behavioural styles of men and the activity levels of both men and women, are reallocated irrespective of their premarital values; only the premarital HIV status is retained. Divorced men and women are 'compressed' to a single 'heterosexual' style, but they also retain their earlier married HIV status. Later marriages reallocate divorced or widowed partners to style and level, according to the menu values, exactly as for first marriages; again, HIV status is retained. The marriage of single prostitutes who continue with their careers is essentially irrelevant to the part they play in spreading transmissible diseases, and entry to prostitution by married women is in practical terms no different from a single woman taking up the profession. For the purpose of the model, and particularly since the frequency of prostitution is rather low, the marriage of prostitutes is not recognized and a married status is not allocated. In effect, they are treated as if single, even when married.

Post-initiation Rates of Partner Acquisition

Each of the three sexual activity levels, in each of the marital states and sexual styles, was associated with an absolute value (a) representing the number of new partners per annum at the age of peak activity. In this context, 'new' refers to partners after the first partner (see Appendix A16). The values were factually based, and derived from the survey data, but are to some degree uncertain. Apart from the internal inconsistencies

Table 17.3

Sexual Styles and Levels of Partner Acquisition

Proportional Distributions

			Levels			
			1	2	3	All Levels
1) Females						
Single Styles						
Selective	0.999	×	0.2	0.5	0.3	1.0
Prostitute	0.001	×	0.1	0.3	0.6	1.0
	1.000					
2) Males						
Single Styles*						
heterosexual (v)	0.950	×	0.2	0.5	0.3	1.0
bisexual/penetrative (vp)	0.005					
bisexual/receptive (vr)	0.005					
bisexual/both (vpr)	0.015	×	0.2	0.5	0.3	1.0
homosexual/penetrative (p)	0.005					
homoscxual/receptive (r)	0.005					
homosexual/both (pr)	0.015					
	1.000					
3) Married Pairs						
Males (× 0.35 unfaithful)						
as Single Styles		×	0.2	0.5	0.3	1.0
Females (× 0.35 unfaithful)		×	0.3	0.5	0.2	1.0
Pairs distributed as products of above proportions, with correlation of 0.6						
4) Divorced, widowed						
Males as single heterosexual	. . .		0.2	0.5	0.3	1.0
Females as single selective	. . .		0.2	0.5	0.3	1.0

*(v=vaginal: p=penetrative anal: r=receptive anal)

within the questionnaires, the evident bias of the samples, and the gender incompatibilities, there was evidence of a rapid increase in rates of partner-change in recent cohorts, pointing towards an augmented future. Behavioural projections are inevitably uncertain. It is even difficult to decide how far the recent increases in reported partner-acquisition rates represented a genuine evolution of behaviour, or how much might have been due to a contrast between recent and well-recalled partners, and the faded memory of more distant partnerships among respondents in the older cohorts. It was nevertheless necessary to settle upon a parameter-setting which would reasonably represent immediate and more distant future behaviour patterns of the population whose HIV-future must be predicted.

Numbers of partners are determined in the model as a complex function of a 'peak' rate modified by age and by cohort loadings, and by changing distributions within the different levels of activity. The survey values cannot therefore be represented as single numerical entries. The choice of values was approached through an iterative series of program runs with repeated re-setting of the peak-activity parameters (a); not only this parameter, but also the age-modifying factors (operating through the Weibull function), and a series of cohort loadings. The process was steered by intermediate print-outs of annual numbers of heterosexual partners taken by males and females, and of reciprocating partners for the different styles of homosexuality. The parameters were reset to balance demand and supply, and at the same time to represent the observed values with reasonable accuracy. Although the model adjusts imbalances between reciprocating sexual behaviours at each annual cycle, we thought it prudent at least to start the simulated activities with the different components in approximate balance.

Reconciliation of the discrepant reports of the males and the females in the samples hinged partly upon the proportion of male activities which had been absorbed by prostitutes; and more importantly, since the reported proportion of prostitute usage was small and perhaps atypical, the proportion which would be absorbed by prostitutes in the general population. We needed an operational decision, if not a clear scientific answer, on two separate questions namely i) what proportion of women are prostitutes? and ii) how many partners do they engage?

The serious difficulties in answering these questions were described in Chapter 15. For the purposes of compiling a provisional set of parameters for the model we had to adopt uncomfortable compromises between the evidence of different studies. We supposed that the prevalence of prostitutes amounted to 1.0 (rather than 2.0) per 1,000 women and that the 'central' number of clients (level-2) was 350 per year. The lower and upper bands offered services at half and at twice this level. After a good deal of trial and error-adjustment, the proportional distribution between the three bands was set at 0.1, 0.3 and 0.6. This results in an overall mean of 542 clients per prostitute-year. This would be sufficient to account for approximately 6.8 percent of the partners of males within the model. This was more than the prostitute encounters to which our respondents had admitted, but less than the estimates obtained from the independent survey of Birmingham prostitutes, or the number necessary to close the reported gender gap. This process of trial and error arrived eventually at the provisional 'standard-set' of values, shown in Tables 17.4, 17.5 and 17.6.

Table 17.4

Annual Partner Acquisition Rates: by Activity Level

	Level		
	1	2	3
Male Singles			
heterosexual (v)	0.55	1.10	2.20
bisexual (vp)	3.0	6.0	12.0
bisexual (vr)	3.0	6.0	12.0
bisexual (vpr)	6.0	12.0	24.0
homosexual (p)	3.0	6.0	12.0
homosexual (r)	3.0	6.0	12.0
homosexual (pr)	6.0	12.0	24.0
Female			
selective single	0.35	0.70	1.40
prostitute	175.0	350.0	700.0
extramarital	0.35	0.70	1.40
Male extramarital			
heterosexual (v)	0.5	1.0	2.0
bisexual (vp)	1.0	4.0	8.0
bisexual (vr)	1.0	4.0	8.0
bisexual (vpr)	1.0	4.0	8.0
homosexual (p)	2.0	8.0	16.0
homosexual (r)	2.0	8.0	16.0
homosexual (pr)	2.0	8.0	16.0

Age-preferences

Age of female partner = (man's age) × 0.65 + 3

Age of male partner = (woman's age) × 0.65 + 8

Sampling range = + − 15% of selected age, with asymmetry factor

Table 17.5

Age Variations in Sexual Activities

Weibull Parameters

	t_0	t_1	c
Single male heterosexual	15	17	1.0
Single homo-bisexual	15	19	1.0
Single female	15	19	1.0
Prostitute	14	18	1.0
Married heterosexual male	15	20	1.0
Married bisexual male	15	24	1.0
Married female	15	20	1.0

$$r = t^c \exp(1 - t^c)$$
where $t = (\text{current-age} - t_0)/(t_1 - t_0)$

Table 17.6

Cohort Variations in Sexual Activities

Model Parameters

Age-band at Year-0 of simulation	Activity-Multipliers
<10	1.80
10-14	1.55
15-19	1.30
20-24	1.20
25-29	1.00
30-34	0.90
35-39	0.80
40-44	0.75
>44	0.70

These parameters resulted in an initial lifetime total of about eight heterosexual partners for both men and for women. This is rather conservative relative to the survey results for the later cohorts, but later calendar years in subsequent simulations showed a steady increase, close to the values observed.

The Reproductive Ratio

The viability of any epidemic depends upon the Reproductive Ratio (R) of current cases. R is the number of new cases which each current case will generate throughout its existence. This is not an intrinsic characteristic of the disease alone, and it depends also upon the social environment. In addition to intrinsic infectivity, it depends upon the numbers of people contacted, and the proportion of susceptibles among them. It therefore varies from time to time and from place to place. So long as R> 1.0, so that each case generates on average at least one other case, then the prevalence and incidence of the infection will grow. If R< 1.0 then the epidemic will decline. The value of R may differ in different sub-groups with the result that the epidemic may be growing in one circumstance and declining in another. In the case of a sexually transmitted disease the reproductive ratio of the disease in an infected female may be different from that in an infected male. This may be because their intrinsic infectivities differ, or because their patterns of social contact are different: or both.

The intrinsic infectivity is the proportion of susceptible contacts who will become infected. In the present instance the practicalities of observation demand that this be stated per unit time of continuing contact, rather than per act of intercourse. The probability of an infective person transmitting the disease depends in part upon this value, but also upon the duration of the infective period (d). For example, an infective man who spreads his contacts among a large number of susceptible women over an infective duration (d) of ten years, and with an infectivity (c) of 0.08 transmissions per year, gives R =0.8. If $c = 0.2$, then R = 2.0. In general, R = cd. However, these values for R are reduced if the rate of acquisition of new partners (a), is limited. At the extreme, if the infected person should remain for the rest of his/her life with a single partner, then he/she can infect a maximum of only one person, no matter how high the intrinsic infectivity; and even a single partner can escape. The greater the number of partners contacted, the more closely will R approach cd. In the case of alternating male and female transmission, with two intrinsic infectivities, c_1 and c_2, the upper limit for R will be d $\sqrt{c_1 c_2}$.

The value of R is important not only for determining the viability of the epidemic, but for determining the rate of decline of a non-viable process. In a sub-stratum in which the epidemic is not autonomously viable, R will determine the number of cases occurring before it dies out. For example, if an infection is introduced to a sub-stratum of the population where R=0.9, then that case will generate 0.90 secondary cases: 0.81 tertiary cases: 0.73 quaternary . . . and so on to R^n. The total cost of a unit introduction will amount here to 10 cases. In general, when R<1, the total number of cases generated by a single introduction will amount to 1/(1-R) cases. A number of small highly-active sub-groups, each maintaining their own epidemics, and continually introducing new infections to groups in which the epidemic is marginally sub-viable, will generate large numbers of secondary infections in these other groups.

Numerical relationships between R, a, c and d are illustrated in Table 17.7. (The basis of the calculations is in Appendix A17). The relative effects of proportional changes in a or in c, differ in different parts of the parameter space. In those parts of the parameter-space with which we shall be concerned, the boxed zone in Table 17.7, small changes in c (or $\sqrt{c_1\,c_2}$) are extremely important; while equivalent proportional variations in a make relatively little difference. For example, if we start with $c = 0.1$ and $a = 0.50$ (the single boxed value in Table 17.7) then a 20 percent increase or decrease of c (a single column either way) results in a near-proportional change in R. By contrast, a 60 percent decrease or a 100 percent increase in a (adjacent rows) results in a much less than proportional variation of R. We should anticipate, both in real life and in simulation studies, that changes in infectivity will have a much greater effect than equivalent proportional changes in similar partner acquisition rates.

However, for a disease with higher values for c, the proportional effects of variations in a are much more important. In each case, however, there is always a critical level beyond which additional increases in a make little further difference. We shall see later that in the case of HIV, rates of partner-change have already passed this level.

We supposed, from a perusal of the original literature and of secondary analyses by others, that the pre-AIDS phase probably lasted about 10 years, that its infectivity was

Table 17.7

Reproductive Ratios (R) for fixed d (12 yrs) and varying a and c

a (partner-acquisition rate)	c (infective transfers per annum)											
	0.08	0.10	0.12	0.14	..	0.20	0.22	0.24	..	1.4	1.6	1.8
0.05	0.72	0.84	0.95	1.04		1.24	1.29	1.34		1.60	1.60	1.60
0.10	0.78	0.92	1.06	1.17		1.46	1.54	1.61		2.20	2.20	2.20
0.15	0.81	0.98	1.13	1.26		1.61	1.71	1.80		2.79	2.79	2.79
0.20	0.84	1.01	1.17	1.33		1.72	1.84	1.94		3.38	3.38	3.39
0.50	0.90	1.10	1.30	1.49		2.03	2.20	2.31		6.37	6.55	6.68
1.00	0.93	1.15	1.36	1.58		2.19	2.39	2.58		9.43	10.03	10.53
1.50	0.94	1.16	1.39	1.69		2.25	2.47	2.67		11.15	12.08	12.90
8.00	0.96	1.19	1.43	1.67		2.37	2.60	2.84		15.43	17.42	19.36
50.00	0.96	1.20	1.44	1.68		2.40	2.63	2.87		16.57	18.90	21.22

Lower viable limit for c is $1/d$: 0.0833

low and constant over much of this time, but that the early period (say the first year) and the late period (say the last year or two) were more infectious; perhaps at twice the basic rate (4,5,6,7,8,9,10,11,12,13). Together with the AIDS phase itself, this would generate an infective period equivalent to about 12 years at the 'standard' rate.

In Table 17 and in the model, the natural history was treated as fixed. It is believed that there is in fact a wide personal variation in the rate at which HIV infection proceeds to AIDS and to death, and the rapid early increase in the epidemic curve has been attributed in part to an excess of 'fast runners'. However, this will be less important a distortion as the epidemic progresses into the forecasting periods with which we are chiefly concerned. We adopted the constancy simplification in the face of pressing requirements to elaborate the model in other respects, and against practical limits of computer space and time, and of programming effort and resource. The main disadvantageous consequence will arise when we try to fit our generated model epidemic curves to those observed in the field. The simulated epidemic will rise less rapidly than the real one. We shall return to this point later.

For countries, regions and classes in which there is a clear heterosexual epidemic, and therefore R>1, the value for c must be greater than $1/d$. For countries where the rate of take-off of the heterosexual epidemic is more tentative or doubtful, then the value for c may be less than or close to this value. For public health practitioners directing their attention to the critical zone between an epidemic which is contained and one which is not, the area of interest is the boxed zone in Table 17.7; also the observation that within this zone, variations in c will generally have more powerful effects than variations in a.

Infectivity Parameters

Several different infectivity values had to be allocated for different modes of sexual transmission, including both male and female heterosexual contacts, and penetrative and receptive homosexual behaviour. The available data on these transmission risks are sparse and unreliable. The values were therefore set only partly on the evidence of available data (4,14,15) and to a large extent upon a process of fitting the consequences of different assumptions to the epidemic patterns actually observed. We develop this process in a later chapter and present here only a set of provisional parameters suitable for initiating this process. The full set of these provisional parameters is shown in Table 17.8. These values are intended to represent mean infectivities irrespective of whether the partners used a condom. The effects of differentiating between condom users and non-users, in terms of their risks, will also be presented later.

Table 17.8

Components of Infectivity: Default Parameters

1) HIV-stages	Duration	Relative Infectivities
1	1	2.0
2	7	1.0 (standard)
3	2	2.0
AIDS	2	0.5

2) Standard transfer-risks by contact-type

infective → susceptible	per annum
female → male	0.02
male → female	0.07
penetrative → receptive	0.80
receptive → penetrative	0.40

3) Prostitute risk

enhancement factor for susceptible prostitutes	3.0

4) Initial HIV seedings (per 100,000)

Prostitutes	50
Penetrative homosexual	100
Receptive homosexual	500
Level-3 male heterosexual singles	10
Level-3 female singles	10

Conclusions

The outcomes of the current epidemic process in this country and elsewhere, and the outcomes of any model which represents it, depend on a wide range of different parameters. They include demographic variables, behavioural variables, natural history variables and transmission variables. Their complexity is such as to make prediction hazardous, and parameter-fitting exceedingly difficult. The demographic data for this country are reasonably reliable. The behavioural data taken from the survey raised many problems of interpretation, chiefly in relation to sampling biases, and are less reliable; but our analyses will show that the uncertainties are unlikely to make a critical difference. Uncertainties about the durations of the natural history stages will result in errors of prediction proportional to the errors in the parameters, but are also unlikely to make critical differences to the outcomes of the model or the real-life pattern of the epidemic.

The truly critical uncertainties and the most serious problems of estimation, relate to the question of infectivity: its level, its variation in time, and its interaction with other sexually transmitted diseases.

APPENDIX A17

Dependence of Reproductive Ratio (R) upon Partner Acquisition Rate (a), Durations of Natural History (d) and Intrinsic Infectivity (c).

This Appendix describes the calculation of the values in text Table 17.7.

1) Infectivity c, is the transfer rate per annum from an infective to a susceptible partner over the period of continuous contact..

2) The new partner-acquisition rate a, will involve $(ad+1)$ partners over the d years for which the disease lasts, each with a mean duration of $d/(ad+1)$ years.

3) The survival probability for one susceptible partner is $e^{-cd/(ad+1)}$ and the probability of infection, for that partner, is $1-e^{-cd/(ad+1)}$

4) The calculations in Table 17.7 suppose that the first partner during the period d was the source of the infection, and that the reproductive ratio is the product of a, and the risk for a single partner. The values suppose that the prevalence is low, and that all partners are susceptible.

Chapter 18 – First Experiments

Figure 18.1 shows the results of a 100-year simulation using the type distributions, the partner change frequencies, the natural history specification and the infectivities, described in Chapter 17 and Table 17.8. These values are strictly provisional at this stage. Their first purpose is to explore and demonstrate the general properties of the model in the circumstances in which it will be used. They are not however entirely arbitrary and were decided after an extended set of trials, similar to the experiments to be described in later chapters.

The heterosexual behavioural parameters are based upon direct observation, but the choice of the biological parameters was more difficult. The male-to-female annual transmission rate for continuing contact was set at 0.07 per annum and the reverse rate (female to male) at 0.02 per annum, both of them attached to the 7-year main (second) stage of the natural history. These values were assigned mainly on the basis of the fitting procedures to be described later, but they are commensurate with those derived or used by other authors (1,16,17,18,19,20,21,22). The one-year first stage and the two-year third stage were each assigned a doubled level of infectivity; and the two-year AIDS stage was assigned half the standard infectivity. For male homosexuals the annual infectivities were set much higher at 0.8 per annum for transmission to the 'receptive' partner, and 0.4 per annum for the reverse. The provisional heterosexual rates are not capable of generating a viable Reproductive Ratio in these circumstances *(see Table 17.7)*: but the homosexual rates are capable of generating an epidemic in almost any circumstance.

For the first experiments, designed to display the properties of the system, condom usage was set at zero. At a later stage we will need to differentiate between users and non-users. The cohort trend in partner-acquisition rates was also set 'level' for these initial purposes. This will be reinstated at a later stage.

During the first ten years of the simulated epidemic shown in Figure 18.1, the numbers of AIDS cases and the numbers of AIDS deaths were determined largely by the HIV 'seedings' with which the process was triggered. It was only after this time that the AIDS cases and deaths began to follow from infections generated through the mass-action forces executed in the simulator. The curve of new infections rose 'log-arithmically' for the first 15 years, after which the rate of increase diminished and was converging on an equilibrium by the end of the 100 year period.

In the early stages, clinical onsets followed infections after an interval of about 10 years, and deaths after another interval of 2 years. As the epidemic progressed, the rate of increase diminished, and the 10-year delay between the curves of infection and clinical onset widened, as did the gap between onsets and deaths. Fifteen years into the

Figure 18.1

HIV, AIDS and Deaths

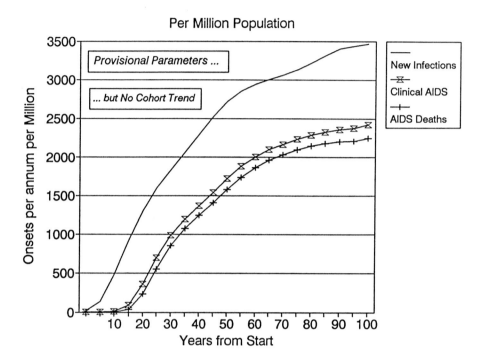

Per Million Population

epidemic, new infections were exceeding current clinical onsets of AIDS by a factor of 10; but by 25 years the ratio had reduced from 10:1 to 2:1. These changes resulted partly from the changing stage-distribution and a reducing mean infectivity. There was also a progressive extension of prevalence into older age groups, with lower levels of new partner contact. In addition, competing causes of death carried off some of the older infected persons before they had time to get AIDS. These changes occurred without any major reduction in the numbers of susceptibles and without any representation, within the model, of biological differentiation into fast and slow runners.

Figure 18.2 shows how new HIV-infections were distributed between different sexual-behaviour groups. During the early years, the greater number of infections (and also of AIDS cases and deaths) were in homosexual and bi-sexual males; but after about 25 years the homosexual epidemic reached a peak and fell a little, while the numbers among heterosexual males and heterosexual females continued to climb. After 35 years, infections in heterosexuals accounted for two-thirds of all new cases, and in the later part of the simulation for about four-fifths.

Figure 18.2

New Infections with HIV

Per Million Population

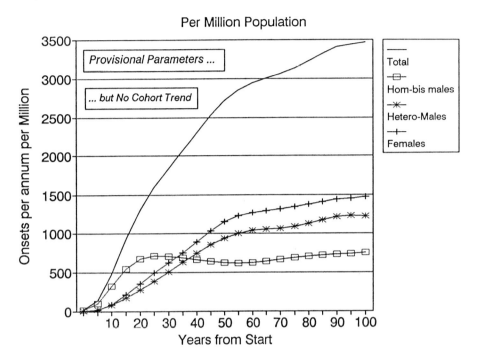

Figures 18.1 and 18.2 record numbers of new events per million total population. Figure 18.3 shows new infections with HIV, in the form of group-specific rates: ie per 100,000 members of the groups themselves. This simulation is limited to 40 years and the graph is set on a logarithmic scale. It shows a rapid increase towards an equilibrium in the higher-risk groups, and a much slower progression among the heterosexual male and female groups. This had been predicted in our earlier model (see Part One). The major contributions of the heterosexuals to the total numbers in Figures 18.1 and 18.2 arise not because their prevalence and incidence are high, but because they are relatively abundant. The slow approach towards equilibrium in the total population reflects the extremely slow approaches in the low risk groups.

Sensitivities to Parameter Changes

Experiments were conducted in which all infectivities were first decreased by 50 percent in all circumstances; and then increased by 50 percent. Analogous runs were

Figure 18.3

New Infections with HIV

Per 100,000 Susceptibles.

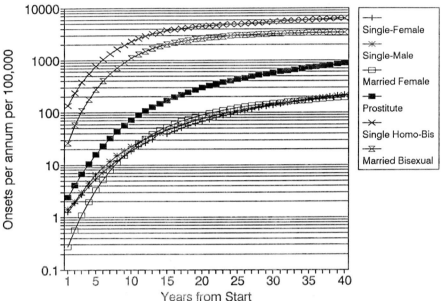

—+—	Single-Female
—*—	Single-Male
—□—	Married Female
—■—	Prostitute
—✱—	Single Homo-Bis
—⊠—	Married Bisexual

then carried out in which all partner-change activities were decreased, and then increased by 50 percent. A further run decreased partner changes more substantially to only 10 percent of their 'standard' values. Finally, both infectivity *and* sensitivity were simultaneously increased by 50 percent. These experiments were carried out using a menu-facility which accepts overriding modifiers for these parameters. All other parameters were the same as those used for Figures 18.1 to 18.3 except that cohort trends of partner acquisition were reintroduced.

The main outcomes of these sensitivity experiments are summarised in Figures 18.4 and 18.5. Figure 18.4 expresses the results of infectivity variations in terms of incidence; while Figure 18.5 represents the results of partnering variations, in terms of total population prevalences. They show that a model epidemic system set up in this way is hypersensitive to infectivity-changes of this degree; but not to changes in partner-switching activity. A halving of infectivity resulted in an effective disappearance of the disease while a halving in partner-changing activity made little difference. A factor of 1.5 applied to infectivity multiplied the incidence (and the prevalence) by a factor of 4, while a similar proportional change in partner-changing activity had little effect.

Figure 18.4

New Infections with HIV

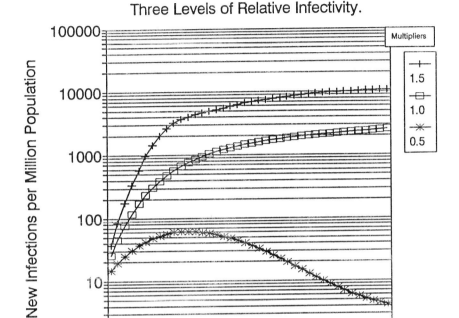

Three Levels of Relative Infectivity.

Years 1 to 40 from Start

The factor of 0.1 applied to the partner acquisition rates – a reduction of 90 percent – did have a substantial effect; but lesser reductions effected little change. It would appear that so far as HIV transmission is concerned, the rates of partner change in the real population are substantially greater than those critical values where small changes make much difference. This conclusion was reinforced when an activity factor of 1.5 was superimposed upon an infectivity factor of 1.5. The outcome was not substantially greater than with the increased infectivity factor alone. We can infer that the real life system will also behave as a natural amplifier with respect to variations of infectivity, and it is probably this which mainly explains the prevalence and incidence heterogeneities in different populations. It also indicates the great difficulties of making accurate predictions from infection parameters whose values are only moderately uncertain; and the equal difficulties of estimating the parameters from the observed rates of epidemic growth.

Figure 18.5

Prevalence of HIV-Positives

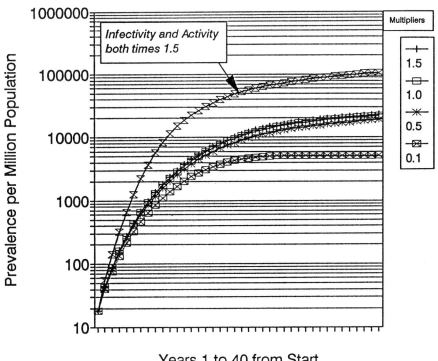

Three Levels of Relative Activity.

Years 1 to 40 from Start

We should not expect all sexually transmitted diseases to behave in this way. Different infections occupy different parts of the formal parameter space indicated in Table 17.7, chiefly with respect to their levels and durations of infectivity. For diseases of short durations and high infectivities such as gonorrhoea, the numbers of partners contacted over short periods of time are likely to play a major part in determining their rates of spread, and of the growth of their epidemics. If, as we suspect, there are important interactions between one infection and another, then the most important mechanism through which high rates of heterosexual partner acquisition assist in spreading HIV, may be through the spread of these other diseases and their indirect effects upon HIV-infectivity (23). This is discussed in more detail later. For homosexual contacts, with their greater infectivities, the direct effects of high partner-changing rates will be relatively important when compared with heterosexual transmission.

Hidden Variations

The simulator was designed to handle a great variety of sexual styles, marital states, and levels and rates of sexual initiation and of partner-changing activities: in all their various combinations, in both sexes: with all of these groups disaggregated by age and by birth cohort. However, we discovered in our survey that there are wide variations of partner-switching activity even within these groups. There are also variations within each partnership-type of the frequency of sexual intercourse, the use of heterosexual anal intercourse and the use of condoms. The last two influence infectivity strongly and directly: the frequency of sexual intercourse probably does: and the partner-changing variations do so indirectly through their effects upon simultaneous infections with other diseases – herpes or gonorrhoea, for example.

In addition, partner-changing behaviour in one person is unlikely to be independent of the behaviour of a partner. A short-duration partnership for one is a short duration partnership for the other: and those who take many partners can scarcely avoid partners who themselves take many partners. That is, partner selection is 'assortative'. Some of this assortative behaviour is handled explicitly in the model design through an imposed extramarital behaviour correlation among married pairs: and by an age correlation between singles, combined with age-varying behaviour. However, the principle probably operates at a more detailed level still, with the important consequence that within each sub-class, those who change partners quickly tend to contact those with a higher risk of being HIV-positive.

Apart from the age-correlation, we had no direct data on the extent of assortative (e.g. high risk with high risk) partner-selection in our study-population: nor of its variation with birth cohort or social group. This is because it was not possible to ask and expect respondents to know about all the partners of their partners. Even if we had obtained such data a practical compartmental model must always simplify real life heterogeneities, and it is doubtful whether variations at such a fine level could be accommodated without sacrificing other important factors. It would also be difficult or impossible to assess how far assortative partnering is neutralised through sexual career shifts: by idiosyncratic individual movements between high level and lower level partner-switching behaviours: and by interruptions in established circles of sexual acquaintances through migration. Together, these opposing or synergistic effects create a difficult technical situation. How do we deal with a phenomenon which is too intricate to measure or to accommodate in a working model, yet too important to be ignored?

The model was therefore equipped with a facility for attaching differential loadings to the prevalence of HIV-positivity in the partners of those exhibiting level-1 or level-3 behaviour. Experimental loadings were designed (when combined with the proportional distribution of the levels) to hold the overall prevalence among all partners,

Figure 18.6

Prevalence of HIV-Positives

Per Million : b-heterogeneity

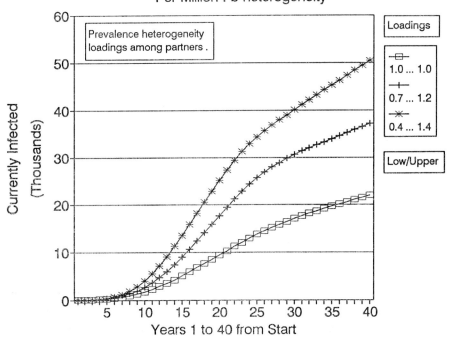

constant. In Figure 18.6 the lower curve is the 'standard', without any loadings, while the other curves are the result of attaching different loadings to the lower and upper levels of activity, as shown in the captions. The effect is to offer the most infective to the most active, a circumstance calculated to increase the number of partnerships having one susceptible and one infective member. The effect is an enhancement of the epidemic. A partner prevalence loading of 1.4 for the upper level of behaviour, and 0.4 for the lower level, increased prevalence by a factor of 2.5 to 3, depending on the stage of the epidemic.

Heterogeneity and Sensitivity

As well as enhancing spread, the hidden heterogeneities in a real population might improve its epidemic stability and ameliorate the more catastrophic effects of small variations in infectivity. The hypersensitivity of the model, as already illustrated, may result partly from the coarse representation of this heterogeneity. A coarsely differentiated behaviour model contains relatively few separate groups, each of which may respond in a dramatic manner to a small parameter change which trips it from a non-viable to a viable epidemic mode. A model which represents more faithfully the multiplicity of small groups of a real population will respond in a more continuous manner. We re-examine this issue later.

Conclusions

The model epidemic, with parameters set at the margins of heterosexual viability or non-viability, is very sensitive to modest changes in the infectivity of the disease. The degree of sensitivity may be less in the real population than within the model, depending upon the manner in which detailed heterogeneities are distributed. However, observations on the gross differences between different countries and different sub-national regions, suggest that these sensitivities exist there as well. The model is relatively insensitive to the direct effects of variation in partner-changing activity around the values currently observed. This may not be true for other sexually transmitted infections, and there is probably an important indirect effect upon HIV transmission which is mediated through the more effective spread of other sexually transmitted diseases, and their effects upon the *infectivity* of co-existing HIV.

The differences between the tentative progress of the heterosexual epidemic in North America and Western Europe, compared with its explosive nature in Central Africa and other third world countries, may hinge upon quite moderate differences in infectivity, the latter augmented by the indirect effects of high levels of partner-switching and widespread unprotected intercourse with prostitutes. Gross prevalence-variations between different countries do not necessarily imply such extreme social or biological differences that a transfer of the epidemic pattern from the one to the other is beyond all likelihood.

These sensitivities of response make it exceedingly difficult to match the parameters of a model with those of a real population. Despite the additional behavioural data now collected, and the progressive development of the simulator, it is still not possible from these first experiments to say whether or not the UK heterosexual epidemic will 'run' autonomously. We may not know whether the infectivity parameters are sufficient to let it do so, until we see it happen. However, once it does 'run', even in a localised region, we could be certain that an explosive outbreak was imminent.

One practical and positive message from these first experiments is that any educational approach which diminished infectivity, whether through treating sexually transmitted disease or an increased use of condoms, or which reduced onward transmissions by HIV-infections through identification and counselling and perhaps segregation of 'positives', will induce savings far in excess of the costs.

Chapter 19 – Predictions and Interventions

Sensitivity to small changes in the estimated biological parameters, in both real and in model epidemic systems, and an uncertain degree of assortative partner-selection, effectively disable immediate hopes of exact prediction. The same factors affect inverse inference: calculating the parameters from the outcomes. They are likely to frustrate estimation of precise parameter values from the observed rate of increase of the disease. The real epidemic may be less brittle than the model system, but future changes in sexual behaviour and drug usage, and the rate of geographical spread, add to the uncertainties of the model/real-life relationship.

The geographical component of the epidemic is not tackled explicitly within this simulator. The national epidemic must be seen as an aggregate of temporally offset growth-curves for different localities; and the pattern of geographic spread, and the successive 'seeding' of different localities, can scarcely be predicted. Sporadic migration of a very small number of infected drug-users, or promiscuous homosexuals, can play a major part here. All these problems apply to any type of HIV modelling.

On the positive side, we now know the rates of partner-change within our society, their variations by age and birth-cohort, the pattern of social variation, and the extent of idiosyncratic variation within particular social groups. Second, we have seen how the application of these measured rates to the model, combined with a realistic natural history and a quite moderate annual transmission-risk, was capable of generating very large epidemics of disease both among homosexuals and heterosexuals. Indeed, the scale of these simulated epidemics was commensurate with observations in third world countries, rather than this one, and more appropriate to an understanding of those epidemics than to our own. Thus, although these experiments supply insights into relative sensitivities to different parameters, and explain the wide international variations, they have not so far provided more than general preventive guidance for the UK.

So What Can We Use a Model For?

The first necessary task is to adjust the combination of input variables to see whether it is indeed possible to reconcile the available social and biological data with the separate components of the epidemic process currently observed in this country. If this proves to be impossible then we shall have to question one or other of the data sets: or else the assumptions which have been built into the model mechanism.

If it proves successful there will still be difficulties, in that the slow predicted rates of growth of the heterosexual component will demand comparative data which will not be available for some time. It is not yet possible to judge whether the sluggish 'take-off' of the heterosexual component in the UK is truly out of step with less conservative predictions.

A second application will be to test the value of different public health interventions. For this, the parameter settings need be only approximately correct. We need an 'operational model', rather than a precise prediction. The choice of the parameter-adjustments is as much a question of prudence, here, as of scientific truth. We need to engineer a marginally supra-critical situation; then, against that situation, to test the control procedures available to us. Specifically, we require a test-bed model in which the homosexual stream of infection is autonomously viable – because we know that in real life it is – and in which the heterosexual stream is set variously, either marginally above or marginally below the level of viability. We shall refer to the latter, the combination of a heterosexual epidemic which is marginally sub-viable and an automonously viable homosexual epidemic, as a 'co-viable' model.

A Co-viable Model

In order to achieve this configuration, the basic behavioural and infective parameters described in Chapter 17 and 18 were modified in two ways. First, partner-prevalence heterogeneities shown in the upper trace of Figure 18.6 (0.4: 1.0: 1.4) were introduced as a standard feature. Second, infectivity was partly controlled through introducing condom usage at frequencies and efficacies suggested by the results of the survey. These latter parameter changes are listed in Table 19.1 and the outcomes of their inclusion are illustrated in Figures 19.1 and 19.2.

Table 19.1

Condom-usage Parameters

Partnerships	Percent usage		Percent efficacy
heterosexual	20	(40)	70
homosexual	40	(60)	75
prostitute	67	(87)	75

() indicates experimental augmented values. The other values were used as 'standard'.

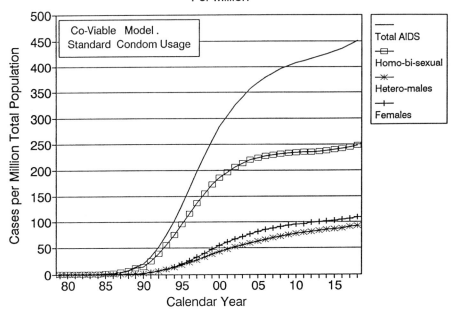

Figure 19.1

Cases of AIDS

Per Million

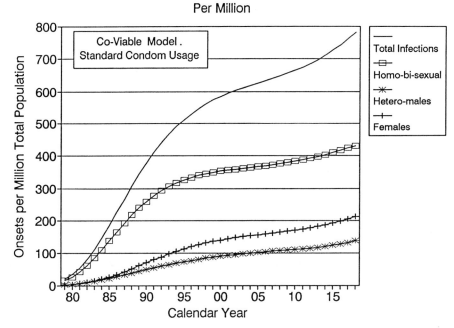

Figure 19.2

New Infections with HIV

Per Million

Figure 19.1 shows onsets of clinical AIDS in different behaviour classes and permits a direct calendar registration against observations for the UK. There were approximately 1,000 new cases of AIDS in 1990: about 18 per million population; so 1990 was lined up with the corresponding incidence on the simulated curve. Figure 19.2 gives numbers of HIV infections, and this permits a trace – essentially a back projection – from the 1980's onwards; that is from dates before the first recorded clinical onsets. The correspondences between the predictions and the observations for AIDS cases are set out in Table 19.2.

This calendar-fitting is provisional. It takes no account of geographical heterogeneities, and the fact that the known cases of AIDS 'belong' to a more circumscribed population than the UK total. Nor does it allow for differentiation between 'fast-running' and

Table 19.2

Simulated and Reported Cases of Sexually acquired AIDS*

Year	Simulated (for 56 million)	Observed UK*
1982	6	3
3	12	26
4	23	77
5	43	158
6	79	300
7	142	642
8	251	757
9	442	842
1990	773	1270
1	1084	1367
2	1839	–
3	2864	–
4	4160	–
5	5671	–
6	7367	–
7	9119	–
8	10890	–
9	12608	–
2000	14234	–

*Small variations are recorded between numbers obtained from different sources. Approximately 90% are believed to be contracted through homosexual or heterosexual intercourse. The latest reports may be incomplete 'slow-running' natural histories. This may be sufficient to account for the discrepancies in the years 1984 to 1987, and the progressive reduction of these discrepancies thereafter. However, the main conclusion to be drawn from this table is that it shows that without too much 'forcing' of the parameter estimates, it is indeed possible to achieve a reasonable mimicry of the epidemic position as it currently stands, both its rate of growth and its distribution between different behavioural groups. It suggests, again provisionally, that the real epidemic is indeed 'co-viable' in character, as in the model.

If the projections of Figure 19.1 represented those for the UK, and if all the Regions followed a synchronous path, they would imply about 21,000 cases of AIDS per year by 2005, and 26,000 per year by 2020. A synchronous epidemic would approach a quasi-equilibrium around 2005; then, as the raised partner-acquisition rates typical of the more recent cohorts extended into the higher age bands, a moderate growth would recommence. Infections in homosexuals would continue to dominate the picture up to the turn of the century, but the proportion of heterosexual infections would then increase. By 2010, homosexual and heterosexual cases would be occurring in approximately equal numbers.

If the growth of the UK epidemic were represented as a series of asynchronous curves, the aggregated growth rate would be flatter and the initial quasi equilibrium of 21,000 cases per year in 2005 might not be reached until about 2015 or 2020. These figures would then correspond with the predictions of our earlier equilibrium model. These numbers cannot be represented as a firm prediction but as a not unreasonable expectation against which we can test, and perhaps later use, the available preventive measures. These measures are considered in turn below.

Use of Condoms

The most striking finding of the experiments represented in Figures 19.1 and 19.2 was the extent to which moderate condom usage reduced the incidence and prevalence of the disease. We have already seen that the introduction of differences in the prevalences of HIV infectivity, between the partners of persons with higher and lower rates of partner-change (assortative partner-prevalence) trebled both the prevalence (Table 18.6) and the incidence of the disease compared with the basic levels shown in Figure 18.2. Yet the introduction of condom usage at the levels shown in Table 19.1 not only countered this effect but drove the total prevalence down to only a fraction of the original: *(compare Figure 19.2 with Figure 18.2)*. The effect was particularly marked among heterosexuals.

The question then arises whether further increases in condom usage, such as might be achieved through educational methods, would reduce the incidence further. An experiment was carried out in which the rates of condom usage attached to the main classes, were each increased by a further 20 percent *(see values in parenthesis in Table 19.1)*. The results of the experiment are illustrated in Figure 19.3.

The effect was dramatic. The initial rate of increase designated at the seeding stage could not be maintained – as shown by the kink in the curve, and the initial momentum was degraded to a short-range trajectory, descending towards the extinction of the epidemic. As with an artillary shell, there is no further force beyond the initial impetus. Allowing for the difference in the scales, Figure 19.3 can be compared with the results for 'standard' condom usage in Figure 19.1.

This experiment was repeated, but this time limiting the augmentation of condom usage to homosexuals and prostitutes. The result, in Figure 19.4, is scarcely distinguishable from the broader-ranging augmentation. This shows that the most effective deployment of a limited health education resource which promoted condom usage, would be towards these high risk groups; and that similar achievements in the very much larger heterosexual group would return only a small additional benefit. It is

Figure 19.3

Cases of AIDS

Per Million

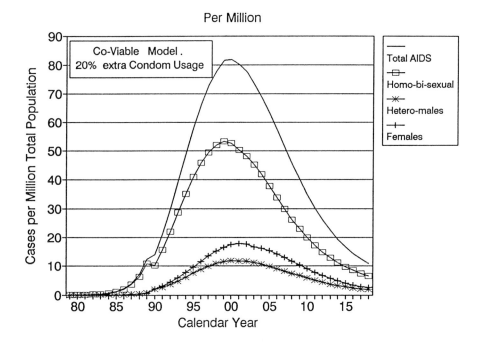

Co-Viable Model.
20% extra Condom Usage

Total AIDS
Homo-bi-sexual
Hetero-males
Females

Calendar Year

Figure 19.4

Cases of AIDS

Per Million

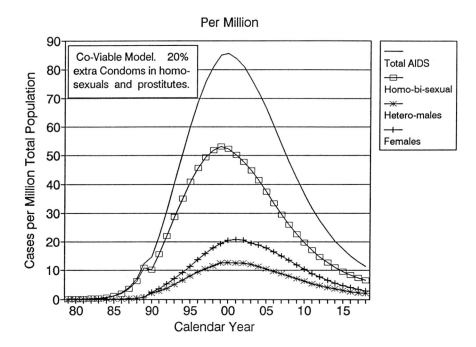

unlikely that this last conclusion would hold true if the transmission rates among the heterosexuals turned out to be rather larger than represented, and if the heterosexual transmission stream threatened to become autonomously viable.

Restricting the Number of Partners

Experiments reported in Chapter 18 showed that the effects of varying the partner-acquisition rates by plus or minus 50 percent were slight. This conformed with the simple algebraic analyses presented earlier. However, the introduction of assortative partner-prevalences, and of condom usage, had possibly modified the characteristics of the system, so this issue must be re-tested. It must also be tested against changes of behaviour which might realistically be induced. The experiment was therefore repeated, first reducing and then increasing partner-change rates by 10 percent across all groups.

Figure 19.5 shows that these changes in behaviour were no more effective than they had been earlier. Prevalence (as in the Figure) and incidence were modified only by

Figure 19.5

Prevalence of HIV-Positives

Per Million

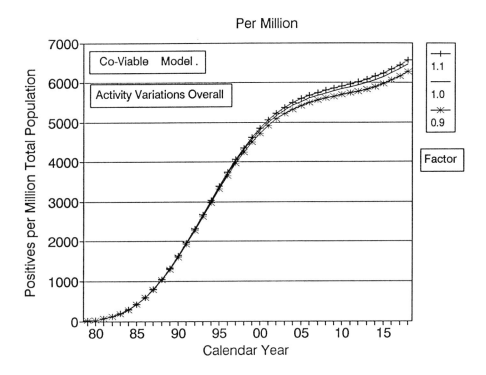

small amounts. The explanation is that with such low levels of heterosexual infectivity, it makes little difference (e.g.) whether an infected person has intercourse once with 100 susceptible partners, or 100 times with a single susceptible partner.

Age Correlations

The breadth of the age differences between sexual partners must affect the evolution of the epidemic. If the age-correlation between partners is high, then a particular birth cohort with a growing prevalence will remain isolated from adjacent cohorts and will extinguish its own private epidemic as its members age and die or withdraw from acquiring new partners. On the other hand, if the age preference is sufficiently broad, then each aging cohort will more readily infect younger people in the succeeding cohorts, and so perpetuate the epidemic.

It is difficult to see any realistic educational intervention which would exploit this phenomenon. The appropriate message for an individual seeking safety is to seek a younger partner, but this is at the expense of safety in the partner. In public health terms, the message is meaningless. A more appropriate public health objective would be to induce individuals to seek partners of ages as close as possible to their own, but it is difficult to see how this could be translated to a meaningful and acceptable message.

We nevertheless tested the effects of varying the age-correlation parameter. The default parameter, at 15 percent, is offered to the model in a form analogous with a coefficient of variation. When the mean partner age has been calculated from the menu-entered regression terms, the coefficient determines two additional ages, one above the mean and one below it, at a percentage-of-age interval, modified by an asymmetry term. The prevalence of infectivity among partners is determined through sampling all three age groups, with a 50 percent weighting for the central value, and 25 percent weightings for the others. The modified experiments used coefficients of 5 percent and 25 percent, instead of the default value of 15 percent. Results for these coefficients are illustrated in Figures 19.6 and 19.7. The difference in the scale is emphasised, in Table 19.7, by including the curve of total infections taken from Figure 19.6.

The smaller coefficient severely curtailed the development of the epidemic, while the larger one enhanced it. The effects were evident among both homosexuals and

Figure 19.6

Infections with HIV

Per Million

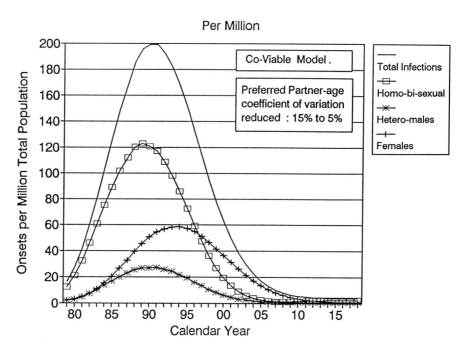

204

Figure 19.7

Infections with HIV

Per Million

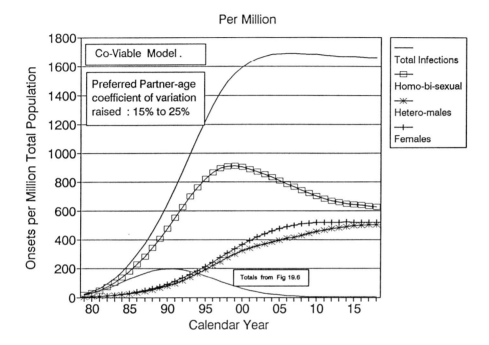

heterosexuals. The development of the age distribution of incidence and prevalence differed under the different conditions, and this is illustrated in Figures 19.8 and 19.9. Figure 19.8 illustrates the way in which a narrow range of partner age-preferences resulted in a 'sweeping-out' of the rising age-specific prevalence, which failed to reinfect the lower age groups. The epidemic eventually collapsed. Figure 19.9 illustrates the effects of a free inter-cohort exchange and a rising prevalence in all age groups. The migration of the greatest prevalences towards the older age groups illustrates the way in which the age-decline of partner-switching activities, the relatively unimportant factor, was overwhelmed by the effects of an increased prevalence of infectivity among contacts. The default coefficient of 15 percent gave results midway between the two.

Homosexual and Bi-Sexual Behaviour

The analyses of condom usage reconfirmed the dominant role of homosexual behaviour in maintaining the epidemic. The question of the degree of dependence of the overall epidemic upon homosexual activity was therefore explored more directly.

Figure 19.8

New Infections with HIV

Per 100,000 Females

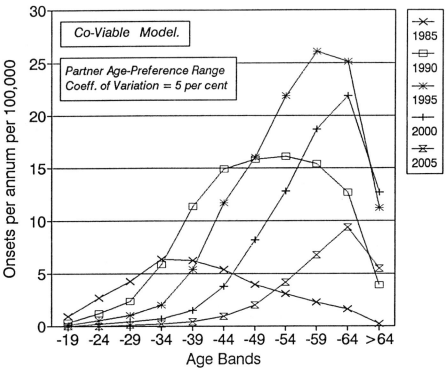

Simulation experiments were conducted in which the proportions of men engaging in homosexual and bi-sexual activity, or the intensity of their activities, were reduced by different amounts.

The first experiment is illustrated in Figure 19.10. All homosexual and all bi-sexual activities in single and in married men were suppressed absolutely. The effect was a total eradication of the epidemic, not only in homosexuals, but also in heterosexual men and women, once the effects of the initial 'seedings' were passed. In practice, this would mean that the epidemic would never take hold. This Figure confirms that a heterosexual epidemic based on the model transmission risks used here, would not be autonomously viable, but could be maintained at a very substantial level through cross-infection from the autonomous homosexual epidemic, through the intermediacy of the bi-sexuals.

Figure 19.9

New Infections with HIV

Per 100,000 Females

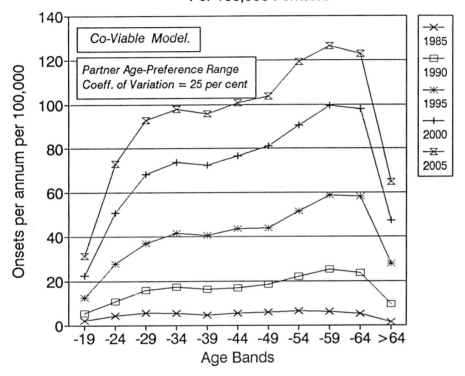

In a further experiment, bi-sexual activity was suppressed in singles, together with all homosexual/bi-sexual extra-marital activity among marrieds. Purely homosexual activity in singles was left untouched. The results are shown in Figure 19.11. Although the numbers of infections were substantially reduced when compared with those in the base-line experiment illustrated in Figure 19.2, and although the distribution between the different sexual behaviour types was altered, the effect on the epidemic fell far short of that shown in Figure 19.10. The explanation lies in the fact that although 'simultaneous' bi-sexuality was abolished, and the means of transfer from homosexuals to heterosexuals apparently cut, the simulator still executed 'serial' bi-sexuality. In particular, homosexual singles still got married. Whether they remained faithful to their wives, or undertook heterosexual extra-marital activities, they took with them into marriage the infections they had acquired when they were single. The heterosexual epidemic in Figure 19.11 is almost limited to females, with only a small secondary transfer to heterosexual males.

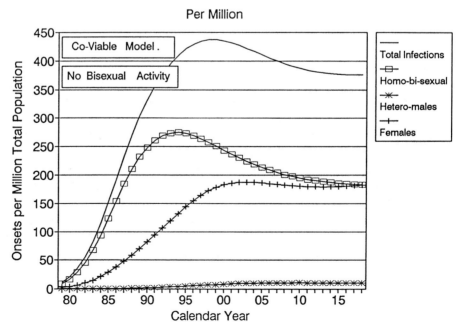

Figure 19.10

New Infections with HIV

Per Million

Co-Viable Model.
No Homosexual or Bisexual Activity
Total Infections
Hetero-males
Females
Onsets per Million Total Population
Calendar Year
0
1
2
3
4
5
6
7
8
9
80
85
90
95
00
05
10
15

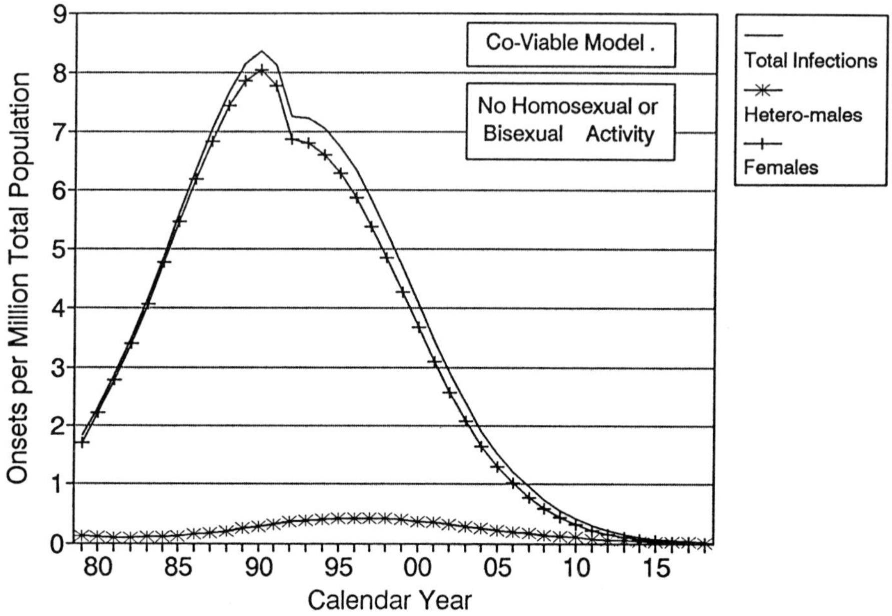

Figure 19.11

Infections with HIV

Per Million

Co-Viable Model.
No Bisexual Activity
Total Infections
Homo-bi-sexual
Hetero-males
Females
Onsets per Million Total Population
Calendar Year
0
50
100
150
200
250
300
350
400
450
80
85
90
95
00
05
10
15

Figure 19.12

Infections with HIV

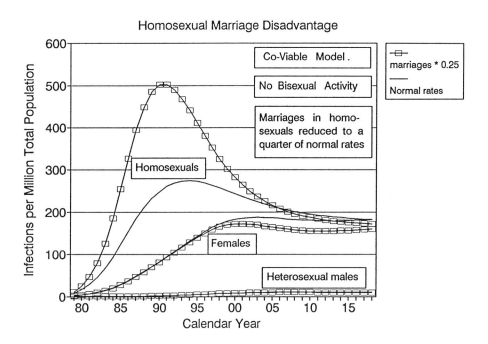

Homosexual Marriage Disadvantage

In a third experiment, similar to the last, the marriage advantage of homosexuals and bi-sexuals was reduced from its default value of 1.0, to the lower value of 0.25. That is, their marriage rates were reduced to 25 percent of those in heterosexual and celibate singles. Marriage was greatly delayed. The results are shown in Figure 19.12. This Figure shows three pairs of lines, an upper pair for homosexuals, a middle pair for females and a lower pair for heterosexual males. In each case the curve for normal marriage rates (the unmarked line) is compared with that for the reduced marriage rates (the marked lines). The results were in some ways paradoxical. The rates among females decreased only a little, and the rates in homosexuals rose sharply, before descending towards an equilibrium level close to the values recorded in Figure 19.11. The initial increase in the homosexuals was due to marriage delay, so that they continued with their relatively promiscuous homosexual activities for a longer period of time. The females incurred the benefit of delayed marriage to these individuals, but the outcome was disappointing because the marrying homosexuals had by then had more time to get infected.

Prostitution

It might be possible, with sufficient commitment and investment, to reduce the scale of services supplied by prostitutes. For example, we might halve the number of prostitutes without altering their individual levels of activity. A trial of such a measure was carried out and the results are given in Figure 19.13. The base line level, with which this should be compared, is in Figure 19.2, although the scales differ.

The results of the reduction were paradoxical. Except for heterosexual males, all the curves increased by about ten percent. The likely explanation is that a new accommodation was reached between heterosexual males and heterosexual non-prostitute females following the part-withdrawal of prostitute services. Overall partner-acquisition rates were reduced, particularly in men, but the rates among non-prostitute women rose. The prevalence of HIV is greater among the simulated prostitutes, but they make greater use of condoms. The risk per contact is therefore small and the part withdrawal of prostitute services was more than counteracted by the greater numbers of unprotected contacts with non-prostitute women.

Figure 19.13

Infections with HIV

Per Million

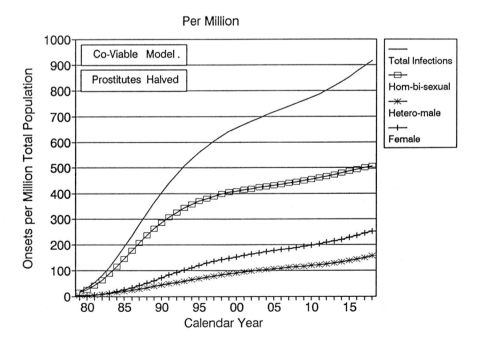

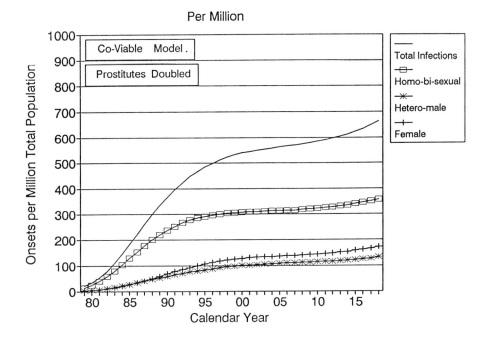

Figure 19.14

Infections with HIV

Per Million

Co-Viable Model.

Prostitutes Doubled

Total Infections

Homo-bi-sexual

Hetero-male

Female

Onsets per Million Total Population

Calendar Year

Further experiments were carried out in which numbers of active prostitutes were doubled and quadrupled. The results are shown in Figures 19.14 and 19.15. These figures are based on scales identical with Figure 19.13 and the base-line comparison, once again, is in Figure 19.2 (with a different scale). In both cases, the epidemic growth was modified downwards.

It is difficult to translate these simulations exactly into real-life situations. The suggestion that increased prostitution would diminish transmission is counter-intuitive, to say the least. The manner in which prostitute contacts are interspersed with non-prostitute contacts is not known, and the supposition that the two compete with each other among the minority of men who use prostitutes, might not be born out in real life. This is an area demanding further behavioural research at a very detailed level.

Extension of Life-span Among those Infected

Some of the drugs available for treating AIDS may prolong the pre-clinical stages of the natural history, as well as of AIDS itself (24). If these drugs do not at the same time reduce infectivity, treatment will increase the prevalence of active infective persons

Figure 19.15

Infections with HIV

Per Million

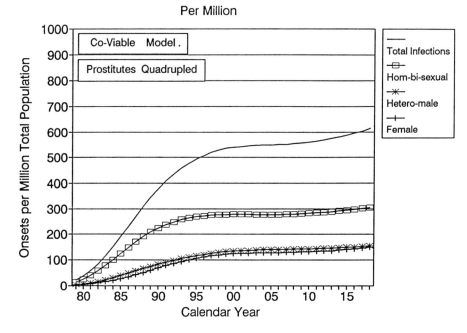

Co-Viable Model.

Prostitutes Quadrupled

Total Infections

Hom-bi-sexual

Hetero-male

Female

Figure 19.16

Infections with HIV

Per Million

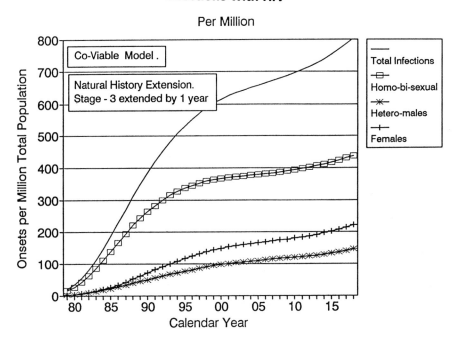

Co-Viable Model.

Natural History Extension.
Stage - 3 extended by 1 year

Total Infections

Homo-bi-sexual

Hetero-males

Females

Figure 19.17

Infections with HIV

Per Million

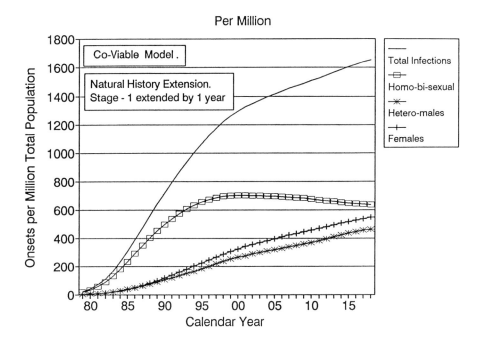

within the population, and thus increase the risk to the non-infecteds. Figure 19.16 shows the result of extending pre-clinical Stage-3 by one year. Despite the augmented infectivity in this stage, the effect was small. This was probably because of the 'wedge shaped' advance of the disease into the susceptible population, as described earlier. Too few of those infected were at this late stage.

A contrasting experiment in which pre-clinical Stage-1 was extended by one year is illustrated in Figure 19.17. Here, the epidemic totals were doubled, and more than doubled among the heterosexuals. It is difficult to envisage any therapeutic interventions which might correspond with this experiment. It would correspond, rather, with a failure of those jointly infected with HIV and some other sexually transmitted disease, to attend for treatment of the latter, thus extending the early period of enhanced infectivity. This is not necessarily a far-fetched circumstance. Fear of discovery of AIDS might inhibit attendance of those with gonorrhoea, or other diseases associated with discharges or ulceration. Educational approaches which raised such fears and provoked such a response, could be extremely counter-productive.

Vaccination

There is at present no vaccine available to control HIV disease. The genetic mobility of the virus is such that the virus genome would certainly adapt itself to the new antibody environment which such a vaccine would invoke, and come to occupy a more favourable antigenic niche. Successive vaccines will become progressively less efficacious as this process takes place, and the immunity of vaccinated individuals will be seen to 'decay'. The basic question to answer in advance, is how best to deploy vaccines with these properties: and probably in short supply.

Initial vaccination experiments were carried out with an assumed uptake of 50 percent, efficacy of 100 percent, and no decay. A first experiment was based upon an offer to males as they reached 18. A second experiment offered the vaccine to females aged 18. No distinction was made between homosexuals and heterosexuals: and none between selective and prostitute women. Rather artificially, the offer was made available from the start of the epidemic. The general properties of these interventions – which is all that such simulations can show – are illustrated in Figures 19.18 and 19.19.

Figure 19.18

Infections with HIV

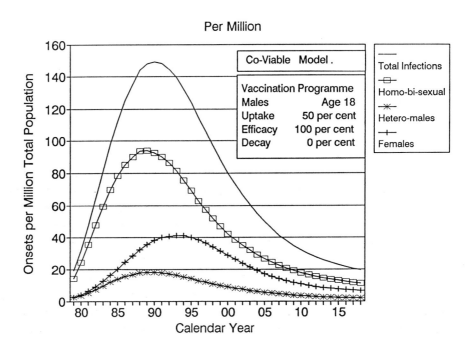

Per Million

Figure 19.19

Infections with HIV

Per Million

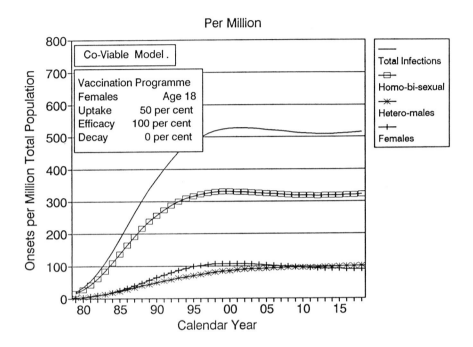

The male vaccination programme was extremely 'successful'. Once the peak level associated with the initial seeding had been passed, the epidemic decayed exponentially to trivial levels, heading for extinction. The female experiment was relatively unsuccessful, reducing the turn-of-the-century totals by about 10 percent. By 2015 the totals among the females themselves had been halved, but this did not approach the decimation attained when the males were vaccinated.

The main effect of the male-directed programme came from the vaccination of homosexuals and bi-sexuals, as shown in another experiment. This was a repetition of that in Figure 19.18 but limited to the homosexual groups. The outcome is shown in Figure 19.20. However, it might be difficult to identify the recipients for such an offered programme and, in any case, vaccination of the heterosexual males did make a useful additional contribution. A further series of experiments was therefore performed exploring the contingencies surrounding a comprehensive male-directed programme; and, in particular, the effects of different decay rates. The results are illustrated in Figure 19.21. This demonstrates the degree to which the protection is degraded as the annual decay rate increases from zero to 20 percent and then to 40 percent. The most striking practical aspect of this result, however, is the substantial degree of protection

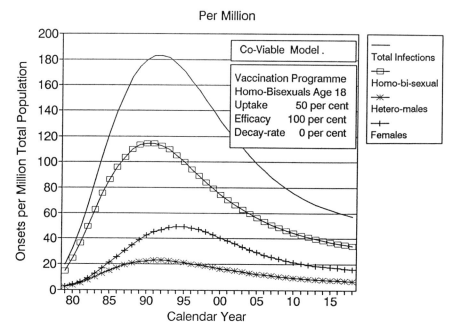

Figure 19.20

Infections with HIV

Per Million

Co-Viable Model.

Vaccination Programme
Homo-Bisexuals Age 18
Uptake   50 per cent
Efficacy   100 per cent
Decay-rate   0 per cent

Total Infections
Homo-bi-sexual
Hetero-males
Females

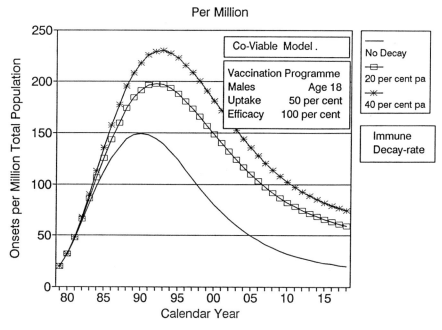

Figure 19.21

Infections with HIV

Per Million

Co-Viable Model.

Vaccination Programme
Males   Age 18
Uptake   50 per cent
Efficacy   100 per cent

No Decay
20 per cent pa
40 per cent pa

Immune
Decay-rate

provided by the less persistent vaccines. A less than perfect vaccine could still exercise a useful degree of control.

The simulator permits the user to nominate the year in which a vaccine programme will begin. Figure 19.22 gives the result of an experiment simulating a 50 percent uptake in 18-year old males and an annual decay rate of 20 percent, but in which the programme is not offered until the year 2000. The effects upon infection rates are almost immediate among the homosexuals and bi-sexuals and in the total population, although the curve representing new infections in heterosexuals is not strongly influenced for another 5 to 7 years. After running the vaccination program for 20 years, the numbers of infections were still declining, and down to a quarter of those in an unvaccinated population, but the full benefits are still some distance in the future. Figure 19.23 is taken from the same experiment but shows cases of AIDS rather than the 'invisible' primary infections. This shows no substantial benefits until about 2015.

Figure 19.24 illustrates a more vigorous programme with 80 percent uptake at two separate ages, 18 and 25 years, but again with a 20 percent annual decay. The benefits, in terms of numbers of cases of clinical AIDS are delayed to roughly the same extent as

Figure 19.22

Infections with HIV

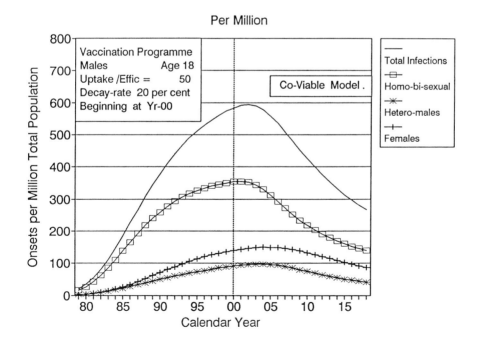

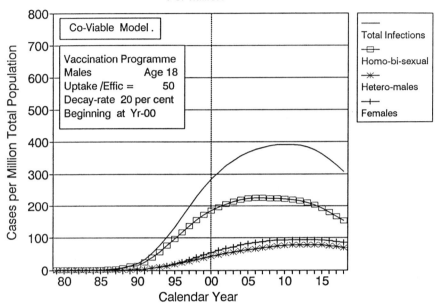

Figure 19.23

Cases of AIDS

Per Million

Co-Viable Model.

Vaccination Programme
Males   Age 18
Uptake /Effic =   50
Decay-rate 20 per cent
Beginning at Yr-00

Total Infections
Homo-bi-sexual
Hetero-males
Females

Cases per Million Total Population

Calendar Year

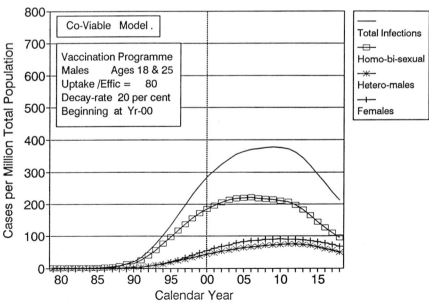

Figure 19.24

Cases of AIDS

Per Million

Co-Viable Model.

Vaccination Programme
Males   Ages 18 & 25
Uptake /Effic =   80
Decay-rate 20 per cent
Beginning at Yr-00

Total Infections
Homo-bi-sexual
Hetero-males
Females

Cases per Million Total Population

Calendar Year

218

in the previous experiment; but when they arrive, they are greater. By 2019, homosexual/bisexual cases of AIDS are only two thirds of those for the less vigorous programme, and the heterosexual cases about four-fifths.

Conclusions

The experiments reported in this chapter are based upon the provisional assumption that the epidemic in this country is co-viable. Its continuity and growth depend critically upon an independently viable epidemic in the homosexuals, combined with a sub-viable level of infectious transmission within the stream of heterosexual contacts. The parameter settings were chosen in order to introduce a realistic degree of heterogeneity of prevalence among the partners of susceptible heterosexuals, and a level of condom usage corresponding with that observed in the sexual behaviour survey. When the model was set up in this way the model showed the same pattern of sensitivities to different parameter changes as those demonstrated earlier for a less refined and less realistic parameter set. The most important finding, still, was that the process was extremely sensitive to variations of infectivity on homosexual or heterosexual contact, and much less sensitive to moderate variations in the frequency with which sexual partners were changed. It would follow that preventive interventions which affect the former are likely to be much more effective than those which affect only the latter.

For example, experiments exploring an increased use of condoms had a truly dramatic effect. This measure alone, if promoted and accepted, can introduce a very substantial degree of control. Indeed, it may be the increase in condom usage reported by our heterosexual respondents – and probably occurring in homosexuals as well – which has prevented the disastrous real-life epidemic explosion which many observers had anticipated. Experimental withdrawal of condom usage created vast model epidemics approaching those observed in third world countries. Educational approaches which effectively persuade heterosexuals to restrict their numbers of partners by any moderate amount, say about ten percent, but without taking steps to reduce infectivity on contact, would be relatively ineffective.

The experiments identified two interventions which might give paradoxically harmful results. The first would be an educational programme which raised the fear of AIDS to a degree which inhibited the attendance for treatment of those with other sexually transmitted diseases. The second would be a reduced usage or availability of prostitutes. Provided that prostitutes continue to use condoms at the levels they claim, and especially if they increase these levels, then a reduction of prostitute services might even induce behavioural changes which would facilitate the spread of the disease. It would certainly appear to be more profitable to concentrate upon persuading prostitutes and their clients to use condoms than to embark upon a probably vain attempt to reduce the scale of activity. Extensions of life span of infected persons through treatment are also unlikely to enhance the spread of the disease by any substantial amount, at least during the growth phase of the epidemic.

Experiments with vaccination confirm that this would be a highly effective measure, even if the induced immunity suffered quite rapid decay. A vaccination programme directed towards young males would be far more effective than a programme directed towards young females. Even the females would be better off if the vaccine were given to the males than they would be if they had it themselves. A vaccine in limited supply would be deployed most effectively among uninfected male homosexuals, if they could be identified sufficiently young; although there is a significant additional benefit from vaccinating heterosexual males. Probably – although not specifically tested in the simulator – the most effective format for a closely restricted deployment among heterosexuals would be to those of both sexes who had already presented with a sexually transmitted disease.

Chapter 20 – Best Predictions

This chapter draws together the findings of earlier ones, and constructs the best specific predictions which the sexual behaviour data and the current epidemic data will allow. It identifies the most important uncertainties and explores their effects upon the predictions. It provides a basis for exploring more precisely the most effective policies for coping with these uncertainties and for limiting the growth of the epidemic in the UK. It supplies a public scientific basis for the formulation of a sound preventive policy, the subject-matter of the next chapter.

Sensitivities and Uncertainties

The chief difficulty in predicting the course of the epidemic, and estimating the effects of interventions, is that those factors to which growth is most sensitive, and on which the accuracy of forecasting depends, are those for which the available estimates are the least certain. There are no reliable measurements of the rates at which infectious partners transmit the virus to susceptible partners, whether in terms of the duration of the contact, or on a per-intercourse basis. Model predictions of growth were extremely sensitive to varied estimates of infectivity, and international comparisons suggest that this is true in real life. Furthermore, it is as difficult to estimate infectivities by observing epidemic growth rates, as it is to measure them directly.

However, this specific sensitivity has an important pragmatic implication. The course of the epidemic in this country is likely to respond to any intervention which influences infectivity. This includes the use of condoms: the use of vaccines, screening, contact tracing and counselling for HIV and other STD's: and quarantine if this should prove to be necessary. Furthermore, all of these measures will be the more effective if concentrated upon high-risk groups, notably homosexuals and prostitutes.

By contrast, measures controlling levels of heterosexual partner-switching, in the region of their current rates and within feasible limits, will have relatively small effects. It makes little difference if the mean lifetime number of partners – currently about eight, and likely to increase by about 50 percent in the next decade – is reduced or increased by one or two. This is a direct consequence of the low transmission risks suggested by current epidemic data.

The risk of transmission is possibly no more than 10 percent per annum from an infected man to an uninfected female partner: and less in the reverse direction. If the mean rate of intercourse is about 100 times per year: then the risk of male to female transmission must amount to about 1 per 1000 acts of intercourse. It then makes little difference whether an infective man has intercourse 100 times with one woman in a year, or 5 times each with 20 women. The first pattern carries a 9.52 percent risk of transferring the disease; and the second, a 9.98 percent risk. If these alternative patterns of activity are restarted in each year of a 10-year natural history – 10 partners or 200 partners over the full period – then neither Reproductive Ratio (0.952, 0.998) quite reaches viability. For an infected female, with a lower risk of transmission, the contrast between the two patterns is even less. A fundamental reduction of partner-changing activity, with a 1000 acts of intercourse between an infected man and one susceptible woman, over the full 10-year period, results in a more substantial change with a Reproductive Ratio of 0.63. The practical consequence of such a reduction are substantial if we consider the full chain of secondary, tertiary . . . etc. cases which follow from a single introduction of the virus to the heterosexual network, but reductions of this degree are beyond all practical expectation.

Two other aspects of partnering behaviour had far greater effects upon the growth of the model epidemic than did changes in the overall average rate of partner acquisition. The first was the correlation between partners' ages. A close age correlation severely restricted the development of the epidemic. The second was an assortative partnering behaviour such that the partners of the most highly active had an enhanced prevalence of infectivity. We obtained no information on this from our survey, or elsewhere, so the manner of its representation was necessarily arbitrary. This limits further the specificity of the predictions which are possible.

Other sexually transmitted diseases with higher infectivities than HIV, respond more dramatically to variations in partner-switching rates. If a disease is infectious for a few weeks, and has a 90 percent risk of transmission on contact, then it makes a great deal of difference whether the infected person contacts none or two or five new partners during that time. This has an indirect but important implication for HIV. The chief effects of higher or lower partnering rates upon HIV transmission will probably operate through altering the risks of these other diseases, thus influencing the infectivity of co-existing HIV. Once more, there is little or no factual evidence from which to estimate the extent of this effect within our population; and again, its representation within the simulator was arbitrary.

Infectivities among homosexuals are greater than among heterosexuals. This conclusion follows necessarily from the fact that the homosexual epidemic exists, while the existence or imminence of a heterosexual epidemic is in doubt. In this elevated infectivity-range we would expect a different balance of sensitivities to infectivity and activity variations. Even here, however, experimental variations in infectivity had a greater effect than did equivalent variations in rates of partner-acquisition.

Homosexual and Heterosexual Transmission

All the predictive exercises showed that the initial dominance of HIV infection among homosexuals will eventually be eroded, and that infections among heterosexuals may eventually occupy an equivalent or even a dominant place. This is chiefly a function of the relative abundance of heterosexuals, and the group-specific prevalence is likely to remain much lower than among the homosexuals. Under the conditions assumed in most of the simulations, only the homosexual epidemic was self-sustaining, while continuation of the heterosexual epidemic depended upon transfers from the homosexual stream.

Under these conditions, we must ask what would be the effect of small variations in the model estimates, or of real life variations, of heterosexual transmission risks alone, without any variation in the homosexual risks. Experiments were conducted to raise these infectivities towards, and then through, the levels required for heterosexual self-sustenance. The male-to-female transmission risk-parameter was first raised from 0.07 per annum to 0.10, and the female-to-male risk from 0.02 to 0.05. The first risk was then raised to 0.15 and the second to 0.08. Figures 20.1 and 20.2 show the effects of

Figure 20.1

Cases of AIDS

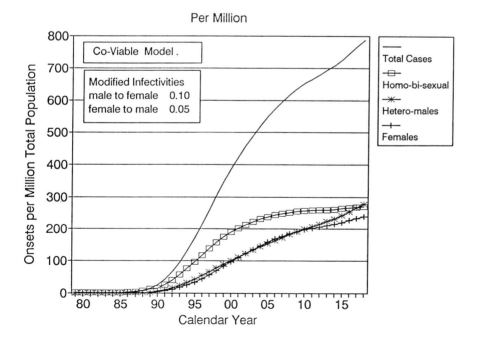

Per Million

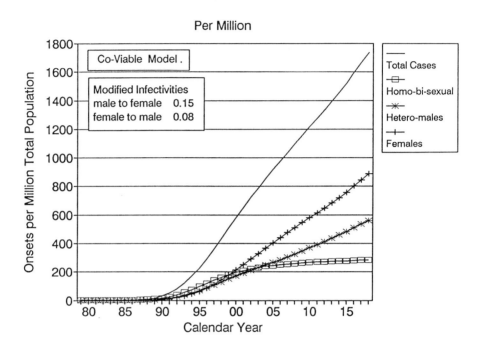

Figure 20.2

Cases of AIDS

Per Million

these changes. The first change raised the total incidence of AIDS in 2015 from 400 per million per annum to 700; and the second raised it to 1600.

Figure 20.3 shows only the heterosexual curves of the last two experiments, together with the effects of yet a further increase in infectivity, now raising the transmission-risk estimates to 0.20 and 0.10 per annum. The non-linear nature of the response in this fraction of the population is now more clearly evident.

Figure 20.4 repeats the experiments of Figure 20.3, but with simultaneous suppression of all homosexual and bi-sexual activity. This new experiment was designed to test the independent viability of heterosexual epidemic in the absence of continuing re-infection from the homosexual stream. This suppression reduced the incidence in heterosexuals in the middle and lower curves of Figure 20.3, to minimal levels. For these curves, an interaction with the homosexual transmission stream was clearly necessary for the survival of the virus. However, the further increases in heterosexual transmission risks (0.2, 0.1) in the upper curves of Figure 20.3, were sufficient to push the heterosexual stream of transmission through the viability barrier. Here, suppression of the homosexual component failed to eliminate the disease among heterosexuals:

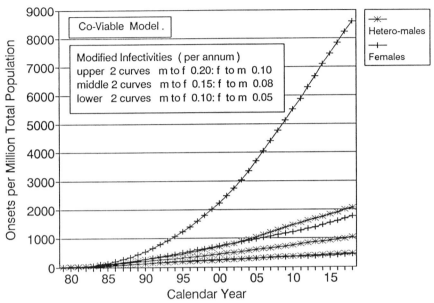

Figure 20.3

Infections with HIV

Per Million

Co-Viable Model.
Modified Infectivities (per annum)
upper 2 curves m to f 0.20: f to m 0.10
middle 2 curves m to f 0.15: f to m 0.08
lower 2 curves m to f 0.10: f to m 0.05
Hetero-males
Females
Onsets per Million Total Population
0
1000
2000
3000
4000
5000
6000
7000
8000
9000
80
85
90
95
00
05
10
15
Calendar Year

Figure 20.4

Infections with HIV

Per Million

Co-Viable Model.
Modified Infectivities (per annum)
upper 2 curves m to f 0.20: f to m 0.10
middle 2 curves m to f 0.15: f to m 0.08
lower 2 curves m to f 0.10: f to m 0.05
No Homosexual Activity
Hetero-males
Females
Onsets per Million Total Population
0
500
1000
1500
2000
2500
3000
3500
4000
4500
5000
80
85
90
95
00
05
10
15
Calendar Year

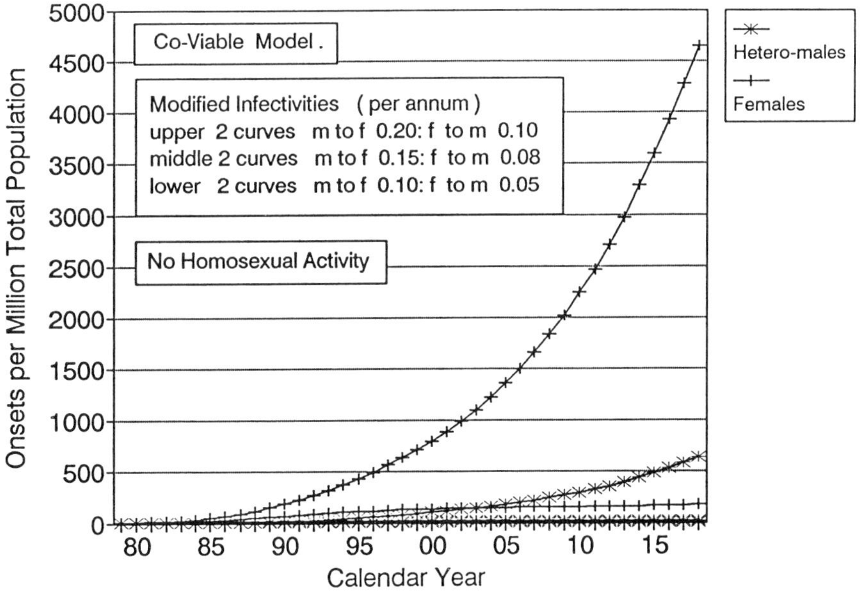

although there was a reduction. A heterosexual epidemic of this nature, in real life, could no longer be contained through measures directed towards the homosexual stream alone. Between the upper and lower values shown in Figures 20.3 and 20.4, the position rests on the knife edge of the heterosexual transmission risk.

Other High Risk Groups

The several high risk groups which contribute to geographical spread, to local seeding and to initial epidemic growth, include female prostitutes, male homosexual prostitutes, intravenous drug users, inmates of prisons, haemophiliacs and immigrants from higher prevalence zones. Our survey yielded no direct evidence on these groups, although there are many descriptions of them, now, within the literature (25, 26, 27, 28, 29, 30, 31, 32, 33, 34). The model was designed to accommodate both intravenous drug users and female prostitutes but the reported experiments have catered only for the latter. Apart from the difficulties in designing meaningful simulation experiments, it is questionable whether any of the other groups could play a unique and critical role in the further development of the epidemic, beyond initial local seeding. Needle-sharing drug users are mainly male, and they and their partners are largely segregated from the remainder of the population. Their more extended sexual activities have effects similar to those of promiscuous bi-sexuals, and for modelling purposes they can be regarded as a component of that stream. There is an important interaction between drug usage and prostitution, but the simulated effects of female prostitution did not appear to play a major role in the dynamics of epidemic growth. Haemophiliacs and infected immigrants likewise contribute to the initial 'seeding' of the population, but are not important to the mechanics of continuity. For these reasons, and because all of these groups are much less frequent within this population than the homosexuals, it is with the latter that the chief opportunities for prevention lie.

Estimating Risk

The crucial question, for Britain, is whether the actual infectivity levels will flip the heterosexual epidemic one way or the other. If they turn out to be sub-viable, and remain so, then the epidemic can be controlled through attention to its homosexual component, without the need to invoke difficult and intrusive measures to control heterosexual transmission. Present evidence seems to indicate that infectivity is low, but the data are not totally concordant and there are at least three disquieting elements. First, the epidemic is not yet so far advanced that we can be sure that it will not 'ignite'. Second, there are sufficient examples of infection having been transmitted heterosexually from one person to several people, to suggest that infectivity is not as low as the current epidemic data seem to show. Third, the determining parameters are continually changing, and the immediate past is not a reliable guide to the future. These changes might include a progressive adaptation of the organism to its circumstances, leading to the evolution of a longer natural history and an improved facility for infectious transfer.

Good quantitative evidence on infectivity is lacking. Many hopes have rested upon the surveillance of haemophiliac male infectives with known dates of infection, and continuing observation of their partners. However, even this is problematical in that these people know their situation and some have presumably taken precautions – condoms, abstinence – to avoid the risk of transfer. Their experience can not be transferred directly to the silent infectives in the general population. There is indeed evidence of relatively high transmission rates among some early haemophiliac cases, in continuing contact with their partners, before the nature of the epidemic was fully appreciated (15). As regards the risk of transmission from an infected female to a susceptible male, we have practically no quantitative data at all. The fact of transmissibility rests chiefly upon anecdotes of contacts with prostitutes, and upon third-world patterns of transmission. This risk, if it is sufficiently low, will constitute the chief barrier to explosive epidemic growth in this country.

Monitoring Systems

Because current heterosexual infectivities can not at present be estimated, and because they may change, they will remain a cause of serious anxiety over the next decade. The situation therefore demands continued monitoring if we are to detect clear early signs of heterosexual viability. This would then demand more vigorous public health interventions than a less imminent hazard would justify. Certain interventions would be difficult to implement on the grounds of their intrusiveness, but also because there are questions concerning their efficacies (35,36,37,38). However, if the epidemic was becoming so virulent that these measures were inevitable in the long run, then the quicker they could be implemented the less draconian they would have to be. The monitoring system must therefore be capable of demonstrating the early signs of major disaster with the least possible ambiguity, and monitoring the efficacy of any implemented measures. The most important model indicator of heterosexual viability was a convergence of the numbers of new female infections upon those occurring in homosexuals. Unfortunately, new infections can not be detected without resort to large-scale repeated linked screening of identified persons. It is therefore unlikely that this will be feasible before such time as the disaster is already evident from other data.

A less precise and less timely but nevertheless useful monitor would be a recurring measurement of the female prevalence of HIV infection. This requires only the screening of annual 'random' samples of women. It does not require recurrent screening of the same women or their personal identification, and could be carried out 'anonymously'. Such results are in some places already available for younger women. Figure 20.5 illustrates the same experiments displayed in Figure 20.3, but compares prevalences of female HIV-positives rather than the incidence of new infections, under the terms of the alternative scenarios. Equivalent model prevalences among homo-bi-sexual males are also shown. Although the general characteristics of the warning signal are evident in these model curves it might in practice be difficult to calculate real-life prevalences among homosexuals because we do not know their exact numbers, or who they are (39,40). In addition, the simulation exercises show that as the epidemic progresses much of the female prevalence will occur in older women, beyond those child-bearing ages affording easy access to test-sera.

Identified cases of AIDS among heterosexuals, and among homosexuals, are of little value for this form of predictive monitoring. The disaster is far beyond the point of effective action by the time that this warning signal arrives.

A third form of monitor is provided by antibody tests in the newborn (41,42). This is a direct and immediate indicator. The test may be positive through transmission of maternal antibodies, even when the infant escapes infection. As with antenatal screening, the main disadvantage is the restricted age band of the mothers.

Figure 20.5

Prevalence of HIV-Positives

Per Million Total Population

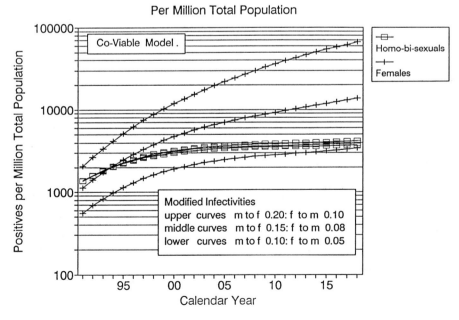

Future Behaviour Trends

The model took account of the recent increases in partnering activity noted in our survey. We cannot tell for how long these trends will continue, or whether they might accelerate. Direct effects upon the progress of the HIV epidemic will not be large, but an increase in other STD's might enhance levels of HIV infectivity and thus promote epidemic growth. It follows that a close monitoring of all STD's – in greater social and geographical detail than that currently available – is a necessary and integral part of HIV surveillance.

The behaviour survey showed an apparent reduction in prostitute usage in the latest cohorts. This may continue. However, it was not clear from our simulation studies that this represented a benefit: possibly the reverse. In pragmatic terms it is less important and less fruitful, to seek to control levels of prostitution, than it is to encourage the use of condoms by prostitutes and their clients. It would of course be useful to identify those who are infected and to isolate them, if this is possible. This is however a difficult and a controversial proposition at the present time, and its justification and eventual implementation will no doubt depend upon the severity of the developing situation.

By far the most important reported behaviour trend, from the point of view of controlling the epidemic, was the reported increase in condom usage by heterosexual men and women. If this has been occurring in homosexuals as well, it will be of even greater importance, although this information was not available to us from our study. The simulations described earlier had set the heterosexual condom usages at the overall levels suggested by the survey, but the simulator did not at that stage allow the incorporation of a trend. A facility for simulating linear trends in condom usage was subsequently incorporated, and an illustrative progression is demonstrated in Figure 20.6. The result of introducing this trend is shown in Figure 20.7. It was sufficient to reverse the epidemic growth and to drive it towards extinction.

Set against field observations, this outcome is probably over-optimistic, and we must suppose that the true infectivity, in the absence of a condom, is rather greater than we had supposed in simulations which disregarded the trend in condom usage. Figure 20.8 redresses this, repeating the experiment of Figure 20.7 but with the addition of a supplementary infectivity factor of 1.1. We are reminded again of the brittle dependency of projections upon small variations in the parameters representing infectivity. With this caveat, however, Figure 20.8 probably represents as serviceable a projection for localised areas of the U.K. as can be obtained at the present time. This supposes no additional effective interventions beyond those in place now. If this result were applied to the whole of the U.K., it would represent about 30,000 cases of AIDS per annum by 2015.

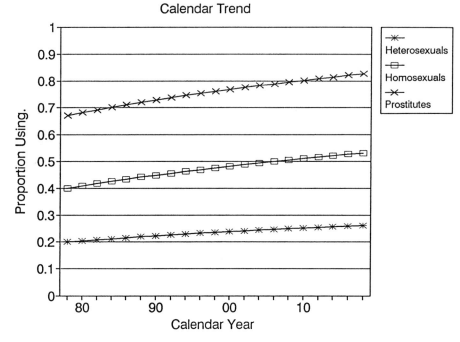

Figure 20.6

Modified Condom Usage

Calendar Trend

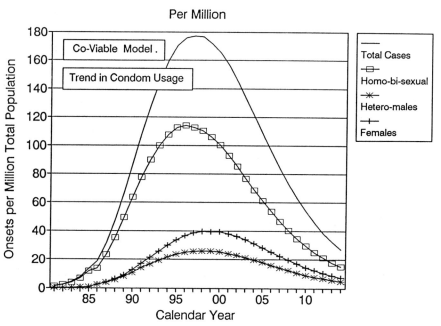

Figure 20.7

Cases of AIDS

Per Million

Figure 20.8

Cases of AIDS

Per Million Population

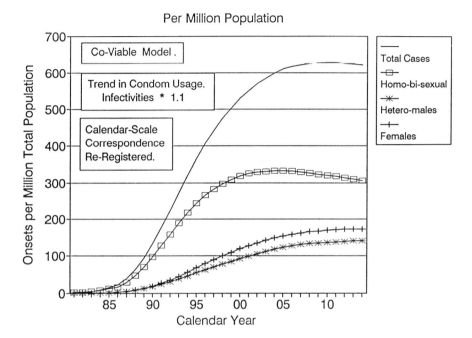

Calendar Year

Figure 20.8 has been re-registered on to the real-world calendar on the basis that current U.K. AIDS data relate only to a fraction of the national population. Most of the reported cases belong to communities amounting to about one tenth of the total. The cases reported in 1990-91 represent an incidence of 100-200 per million of this limited source population, rather than the 18 per million when based on the whole country. Curves of this general form, delayed by a few years, probably represent serviceable projections for other regions as well; and an aggregate of these offset curves would represent a reasonable future for the whole of the U.K. The aggregate curve will be less steep than individual local curves, as represented in Figure 20.8 but the eventual incidence and prevalence would be similar. In aggregate, for the whole of the U.K., such a pattern would represent about 30,000 cases of AIDS per annum by about 2030. This is similar to the predictions of our earlier equilibrium model.

Figure 20.9 shows the model prevalence of HIV positives, per 100,000, in the three sub-classes shown in Figure 20.8: together with another curve for female prostitutes. The homosexuals settled out with a prevalence a little over 20 percent: the prostitutes a little over one percent: and the male and female heterosexuals at about half of this level. To complete the picture, Figure 20.10 gives future frequencies of AIDS deaths per 100,000 per annum, in the same groups.

Figure 20.9

Prevalence of HIV-Positives

Per 100,000 in Each Class

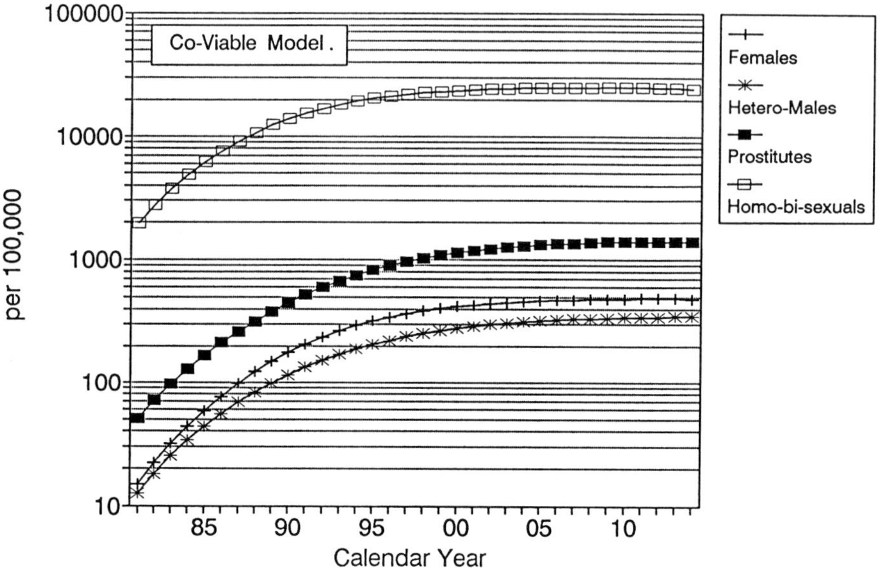

Figure 20.10

AIDS Deaths

Per 100,000 per Annum in Each Class

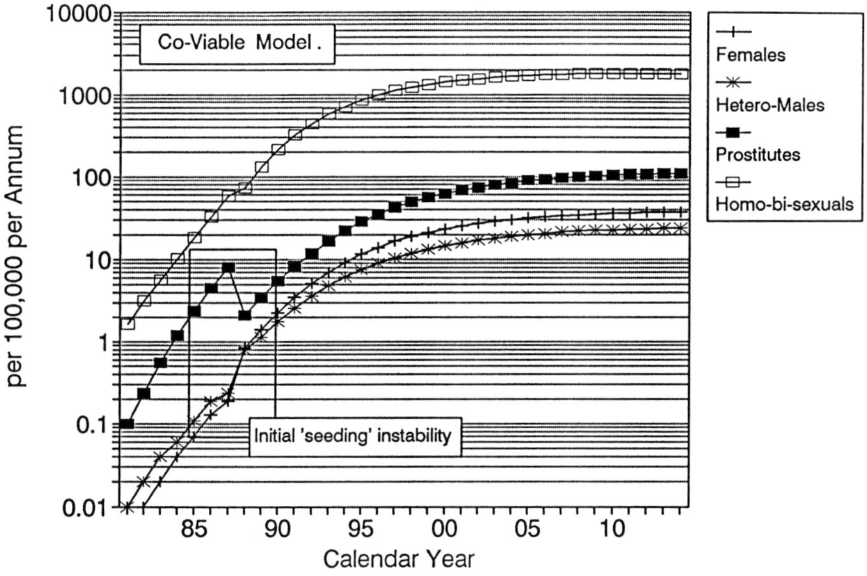

Conclusions

Numerical predictions of HIV infections and of AIDS in the UK depend critically upon current estimates of infectivity on contact between infective and susceptible persons. They depend also upon future trends in infectivity, for which the two most cogent factors are a) changes in the use of condoms by heterosexuals, homosexuals and prostitutes, and b) the extent to which increasing partnering frequencies will raise the incidence of other sexually transmitted diseases such as gonorrhoea and herpes, with secondary effects upon the infectivity of concurrent HIV. It is unclear, and likely to remain so for some time, whether the heterosexual component of the HIV epidemic will enter a self-viable mode, or whether it will continue to depend for its progression – as it appears at present – upon the concurrent homosexual epidemic, and upon transfers from homosexuals to heterosexuals. If it should continue in a dependent mode, then the size of the epidemic will depend mainly upon the extent and frequency of homosexual behaviour: especially the numbers practising anal intercourse, the numbers of their partners and the frequency of condom usage. Using the estimates entered to our simulator, the total AIDS epidemic will probably progress slowly towards a total of 30,000 cases per annum by 2030, although the outcome could very readily be twice or half this number; and lower still if condom usage increases further. However, if the heterosexual epidemic should enter a self-viable mode, as it has in other countries, then the epidemic could expand to reach demographically significant levels.

Chapter 21 – Necessary Policies

In this chapter we identify two broad technical conclusions to be drawn from the studies already described. We then proceed to identify the chief necessary components of a preventive strategy, and the scientific guidelines which govern their design and implementation.

Technical Conclusions

The first technical conclusion is that long-term numerical projections based upon simulation of the sexual transfer of HIV, and upon available data, can not yet be regarded as dependable. Widely varying outcomes follow upon minor adjustments of sensitive parameters. The main present advantage of the approach is that it displays the specific sources of the errors, and their likely range, and it offers scope for improvement as the data-uncertainties are narrowed.

The second technical conclusion is that the immediate problems of predicting the course of the epidemic are no longer issues of methodological refinement, but problems of measuring real life parameters. The most important are the current frequencies and levels of homosexual behaviour throughout the country, infectivities on contact between heterosexuals, assortative partnering behaviours, rates and patterns of geographical spread, and continuing and future trends in heterosexual partnering frequencies and in the use of condoms. Improved modelling methods will not solve these primary difficulties. The most immediate requirement, necessary for any appraisal of the likelihood of a disastrous self-viable heterosexual epidemic, is for improved estimates of infectivity within heterosexual partnerships.

Policy Guidance

So far as policy guidance is concerned, the first major conclusion is that preventive measures which influence infectivity are likely to be successful, while others are not. It is far more important to increase the use of condoms, to identify and contain the activities of identified infectives, and to trace and treat other sexually transmissible diseases: than to try to influence the rates at which heterosexual partners are switched, or to reduce the numbers and activities of prostitutes (43,44). Heterosexual switching-activity in the current adult population is already far beyond those critical levels where attainable restraint would make much difference. These activities are in any case increasing further: and have been doing so in the face of extensive educational programmes aimed towards the contrary.

The second policy guideline to be drawn from these experiments is that the main current public health investment should still be directed towards the prevention of homosexual transmission. It is here that the greater part of the infections are occurring: and the heterosexual epidemic still depends more upon transfers from the homosexual infection pool than upon transfers between heterosexuals themselves. This may not continue indefinitely. For the time being, however, any measure or advice which limits the proportion of men engaging in homosexual anal intercourse, or limits infectivity, or restricts the activities of the more promiscuous or of the HIV-positives, will have profound effects not only upon the risks to the participants themselves, but also to the rest of the population.

A third main component of a preventive policy must be an attempt to limit transfer from the homosexual transmission stream to the heterosexuals through simultaneous or serial bi-sexuality. Even if this transmission fails to trigger an independently viable heterosexual epidemic, the chain of secondary and subsequent infections which follows such transfers is still a major public health problem and may become responsible for many deaths each year. Simulation experiments showed that it was not sufficient to control the activities of current bi-sexuals, and that a major part of the transmission was effected through marriage, or non-marital female partnering, by ex-homosexuals. This demands strong and explicit advice that previous homosexuals – as well as current homosexuals – should have an HIV test before taking up any heterosexual partnership. Those infected should be advised unequivocally that they should not marry or take female partners. Ways should be sought to reduce present disincentives to HIV testing.

A fourth necessary component of the preventive policy must be to develop a system for identifying infectives. The main routes are through tracing contacts of those known to have been infected, and through screening. Screening should be offered specifically to those at high risk, including those with other STD's, drug addicts and prison inmates; to those, such as blood donors, who present a high risk to others; and to those from whom blood is collected for some other purpose such as antenatal care or hospital treatment. However, it should also be offered readily to others who ask for it. Public statements that screening will not be countenanced for this disease should be explicitly withdrawn as should the blanket requirement for anonymity of testing (45). It is indefensible and unethical that both the subject and his/her sexual contacts and medical attendants should be denied the possibility of taking appropriate precautions to prevent further passage of the virus, or receiving the benefit of new treatments as they are developed.

The fifth necessity must be to establish a system for reviewing the current status of the epidemic on a continuing basis, especially with respect to assessing the current and imminent need for intrusive control procedures such as selective compulsory testing or even quarantine. A general application of such direct interventions is unlikely to be acceptable politically, professionally, or socially, unless the hazards are shown to be extreme. Their justification (or otherwise) will have to be argued on the demonstrated magnitude of the hazard; in effect, on the likelihood and imminence of the heterosexual epidemic running out of control. We elaborate on this requirement in the next section.

The Review Process

This will demand a major purpose-orientated surveillance programme of much wider scope than the current system, and going beyond the present purposes of supplying simple statistical returns of cases of AIDS. Epidemiological surveillance will be required at local as well as at national levels and will include recurring statements of the extent and yields of screening programmes and contact-tracing processes. It will include detailed statements – based on follow-up of identified cases – of the risk-groups and ages affected, the sources of infection so far as they can be ascertained, and detailed geographical distributions. Available epidemiological traces of the progress of the disease within the population will effectively be limited to serial prevalences of HIV infection in young females attending for maternity care and in older persons of both sexes attending hospital, in those attending for treatment of sexually transmitted diseases, and numbers of cases of clinical AIDS, chiefly in homosexual males.

The assembly of these data will be difficult, but their interpretation even more so. The signal representing an imminent heterosexual 'breakout' would be a high and rising ratio between the female prevalences and the numbers of cases in homosexual males. However, the prevalence data will suffer from various forms of bias (46), including age bias, while the reported cases in homosexual males will have no known denominator to which they can be related. The measures are also dimensionally non-commensurate, one being a measure of a state, and the other a count of events (47). The functional and temporal relationships between the two traces are not easily defined, and a simple ratio between the two values in a single year is not necessarily meaningful.

Monitoring techniques will have to be developed in situ by those in direct contact with the data and the data assembly processes. The temporal relationships between the AIDS onset data and the HIV prevalence data will probably shift as the epidemic evolves. The AIDS onsets follow a primary HIV infection after a varying interval of five to fifteen years, lengthening as the epidemic progresses. The female prevalences represent mid-course frequencies of a diminishing chain of primary and subsequent transfers of infection, following on from the initial event in a bi-sexual male. The difficulties of direct interpretation of the ratio between the two are well illustrated in Figure 21.1. It would be difficult from the three alternative traces of prevalence in females, in the early years, to say which, if any, represented a course to disaster. The small numbers of cases detected by screening programmes, in these early years, would add a further degree of uncertainty.

Figure 21.2 seeks a more instructive format of presentation. The curves for female and homosexual morbidity are brought into parallel apposition through the use of two graphical 'tricks'. First, the prevalence data are calculated in relation to the numbers of eligible women rather than the total population, and are matched against the AIDS cases for the previous year; and, second, the two curves of increase are set on different logarithmic scales. The prevalence is set upon a two-cycle scale and the incidence upon a four-cycle scale. This is a purely empirical device, with no detailed justification in terms of a defined functional relationship between the different curves.

Figure 21.3 carries these manipulations one stage further, setting out the relationships between the two variables upon a double logarithmic x-y plot. The lower curve represents the 'standard infectivities' as used in Figure 21.2; while the other curves

Figure 21.1

Prevalence of HIV+ Females

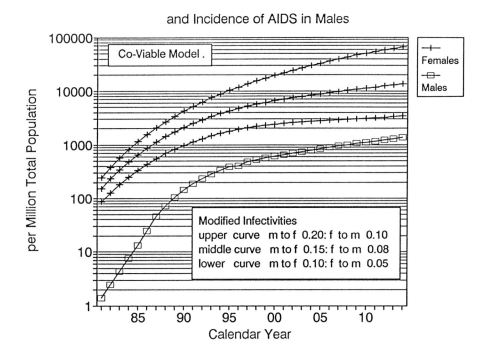

and Incidence of AIDS in Males

Figure 21.2

Stability-monitor

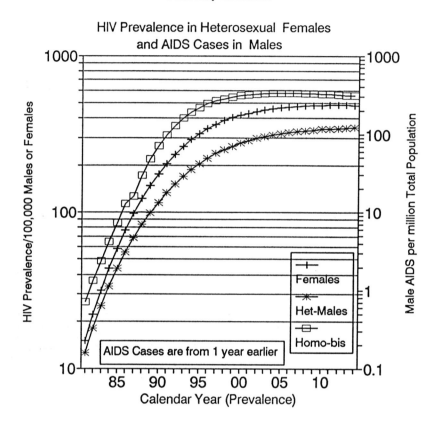

HIV Prevalence in Heterosexual Females
and AIDS Cases in Males

represent the relationships for the progressively increased heterosexual infectivities represented earlier in Figure 21.1. Figure 21.4 is derived from Figure 21.3 and suggests a general format through which these monitoring activities might be pursued and through which particular populations could be tracked.

Techniques for local tracing and projection, based on these principles, will require much additional development if they are to provide reliable guidance. For example, the exact positions of the 'tram-lines' in Figure 21.4 can not be prescribed in advance for any particular community, depending as they do upon the local prevalences, levels and styles of homosexual and bi-sexual behaviour within the given population. These developments will require the establishment of research-groups capable of mounting the necessary epidemiological skills, in control of their data sources, and therefore holding direct preventive responsibilities. These lessons have already been learned and acted upon in other countries.

Figure 21.3

Stability-monitor

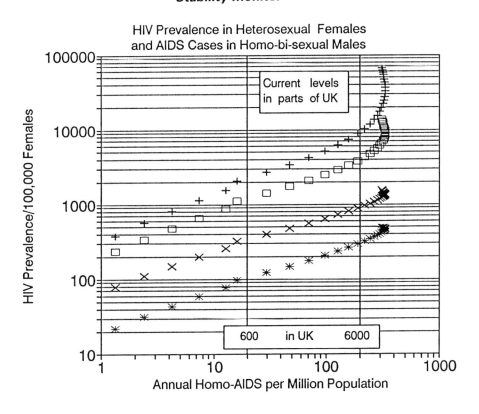

HIV Prevalence in Heterosexual Females
and AIDS Cases in Homo-bi-sexual Males

Detailed data analyses, and a trace of individual transmissions, will be required in geographically localised zones. Geographically aggregated data might obscure sharp localised changes and hide the evidence of an imminent heterosexual breakout. Those responsible for monitoring the epidemic will therefore require the same confidential access to ages, addresses and identities (to recognise duplicate reporting) as those responsible for contact-tracing and counselling.

The last main component of a continuing review process will be a monitor of the styles and the levels of sexual behaviour within each local area. This will be based largely upon recurring sample studies using direct interviews or anonymous questionnaires, or even telephone interview. The most important points of information will relate to changes in the use of condoms by homosexual and heterosexual males and females, including prostitutes; levels of needle-sharing drug abuse; and changes in the prevalence of homosexual and bisexual activity – especially anal intercourse – in different localities.

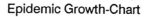

Figure 21.4

Stability-monitor

Epidemic Growth-Chart

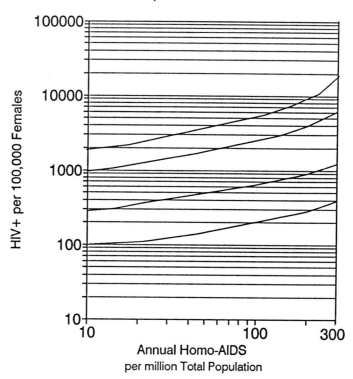

The Control Environment

For all these reasons, a serious attempt should be made to bring the development of the preventive services, the continuing research on which the development depends, and the managerial and professional responsibilities for the control of the epidemic, within a unified framework. Interventions should be designed and conducted under direct scientific guidance within a competent, accountable and adequately resourced preventive organisation, which incorporates responsibilities for research and monitoring alongside those for field control. This public health problem is sufficiently important to demand that the organisation of the service should respond to the specific needs of the situation: rather than that the choice and implementation of the control measures should be constrained by current administrative mechanics.

The concept that research can be done first and put into practice later, as with clinical procedures, is entirely inappropriate to situations of this kind. As with other preventive programmes such as screening for cancer of the breast or cancer of the cervix, the scale and the operational character of the necessary research cannot easily be contained within the context of research-contracts to Universities and Research Councils working separately from a Public Health Service. Nor can a Public Health Service which lacks any central structure or unified staffing, or any specific resource allocation for its operations, or an address or a telephone number – or indeed any legal or titular or institutional existence – use or commission this kind of research.

These are familiar points which have been made repeatedly by public health researchers and public health practitioners over several decades. There is some recent evidence of a beneficial change of attitude at local levels, in an improved acceptance of scientific findings offering guidance for service planning and institutional management, but it is still difficult to recognize the prospect of an adequate response to global problems which extend beyond the boundaries of local Health Authorities.

We have restated the technical and administrative necessities here only because the points made remain obstinately true, because the message is still unheard, and because the hazards attendant upon a continued disregard of public health needs in relation to the AIDS epidemic are likely to be great indeed.

References

1. Stigum H., Gronnesby J.K., Magnus P., Sundet J.M. and Bakketeig L.S. (1991) 'The Potential for spread of HIV in the Heterosexual Population in Norway: A Model Study'. *Statistics in Medicine* **10**: 1003-1023.

2. Koch M.G. and Velch U. *AIDS spread, simulations and projections*. Project Study. Angewandte Computer Software GmbH, Munich 1987.

3. Gonzalez J.J., Koch M.G., Dorner D., L'age-Stehr J., Myrtveit M. and Vavik L. (1988) 'The prognostic analysis of the AIDS epidemic: mathematical modelling and computer simulation' In: *Statistical Analysis and Mathematical Modelling of AIDS*. Eds. J.C. Jager and E.J. Ruitenberg. New York 1988.

4. Anderson R.M. (1988) 'The Epidemiology of HIV Infection: Variable Incubation Plus Infectious Periods and Heterogeneity in Sexual Activity'. *J.R. Statist. Soc.* **151**: 66-98.

5. Medley G.F., Anderson R.M., Cox D.R., Billard L. (1987) 'Incubation Period of AIDS in patients infected via blood transfusions'. *Nature* **328**: 719-721.

6. Pederson C., Nielsen C.N. and Vestergaard B.F., Gerstoft J., Krogsgaard K. and Nielson J.O. (1987) 'Temporal relation of antigenaemia and loss of antibodies to core antigens to development of clinical disease in HIV infection'. *Brit. Med. J.* **295**: 567-569.

7. Rezza G., Lazzarin A., Angarano G., Sinicco A., Pristera R., Ortona L., Barbanera M., Gafa S., Tirelli U., Salassa B., Ricchi E., Aiuti F. and Menniti-Ippolito F. (1989) 'The natural history of HIV infection in intravenous drug users: risk of disease progression in a cohort of seroconverters'. *Current Science*. **3**: 87-90.

8. Taylor J.M.G., Schwartz K. and Detels R. (1986) 'The Time from Infection with Human Immunodeficiency Virus (HIV) to the Onset of AIDS'. *J. Inf. Dis.* **154**: 4, 694-697.

9. Biggar R.J., Melby M., Ebbesen P., Alexander S., Nielsen J.O. Sarin P. and Faber V. (1985) 'Variation in human T lymphotropic virus III (HTLV-III) antibodies in homosexual men: decline before onset of illness related to Acquired Immune Deficiency Syndrome (AIDS)'. *Brit. Med. J.* **291,** 997-998.

10. Moss A.R. and Bacchetti P. (1989) 'Natural history of HIV infection' Editorial review. *Current Science* **3**: 55-61.

11. Darby S.C., Doll R. and Thakrar B. (1990) 'Time from infection with HIV to onset of AIDS in patients with haemophilia in the U.K.'. *Statistics in Medicine* **9**: 681-689.

12. Taylor J.M.G., Munoz A., Bass S.M., Saah A.J., Chmiel J.S. and Kingsley L.A. (1989) 'Estimating the Distribution of times from HIV seroconversion to AIDS using multiple imputation'. *Statistics in Medicine* **9,** 505-514.

13. Gonzalez J. and Koch M. (1986) 'Analysis of AIDS and the Anciennity Distribution of AIDS Patients'. *AIDS-Forschung (AIFO)* **11,** 621-630.

14. Peterman T.A., Stoneburner R.L., Allen J.R., Jaffe H.W. and Curran J.W. (1987) 'Risk of Human Immunodeficiency Virus transmission from heterosexual adults with transfusion-associated infections'. *J. Amer. Medical Assoc.* **259**: 55-58.

15. Jones P., Hamilton P.J., Bird G., Fearns M., Oxley A., Tedder R., Cheingsong-Popov R. and Codd A. (1985) 'AIDS and haemophilia: morbidity and mortality in a well defined population'. *Brit. Med. J.* **291**: 695-699.

16. Peterman T.A., Stoneburner R.L., Allen J.R., Jaffe H.W. and Curran J.W. (1988) 'Risk of human immunodeficiency virus transmission from heterosexual adults with transfusion-associated infections'. *J. Amer. Med. Soc.* **259**: 55-58.

17. Medley G.F., Anderson R.M., Cox D.R. and Billard L. (1987) 'Incubation period of AIDS in patients infected via blood transfusion'. *Nature* **328**: 719-721.

18. Van der Ende M.E., Rothbarth P. and Stibbe J. (1988) 'Heterosexual transmission of HIV by haemophiliacs'. *Brit. Med. J.* **297**: 1102-1103.

19. Johnson A.M. (1988) 'Heterosexual transmission of human immunodeficiency virus'. *Brit. Med. J.* **296,** 1017-1020.

20. Johnson A.M. and Laga M. (1989) 'Heterosexual transmission of HIV', *AIDS 2 Suppl 1*, S49-S56.

21. Johnson A.M. (1988) 'Social and Behavioural Aspects of the HIV Epidemic – A Review'. *J. Roy. Stat. Soc.* **151,** 99-114.

22. Van Druten J.A.M. and Reintjes A.G.M. (1990) 'HIV Infection Dynamics and Intervention Experiments in Linked Risk Groups'. *Statistics in Medicine* **9,** 721-736.

23. Pepin J., Plummer F.A., Brunham R.C., Piot P., Cameron D.W. and Ronald A.R. (1988) 'The interaction of HIV infection and other sexually transmitted diseases: an opportunity for intervention'. *AIDS* **3** 3-9.

24. Ranki A., Mattinen S., Yarchoan R., Broder S., Ghrayeb J., Lahdevirta J. and Krohn K. (1988) 'T-cell response towards HIV in infected individuals with and without zidovudine therapy, and in HIV-exposed sexual partners'. *Current Science* **3**: 63-69.

25. DOH (1989) *Evaluation of syringe exchange schemes.* Circular EL(89) P/81.

26. Stimson G.V., Alldritt L., Dolan K. and Donoghue M. (1989) *Syringe-Exchange schemes in England and Scotland: Evaluating a New Service for Drug Users.* AIDS: Social Representations, Social Practices, London. The Falmer Press.

27. British Medical Association Foundation for AIDS (1989) *Preventing the spread of HIV through shared needles and syringes.* No. 5 of a series of 'Parliamentary Fact-Sheets'.

28. Donoghoe, M.C., Stimson G.V. and Dolan K.A. (1989) 'Sexual Behaviour of injecting drug users and associated risks of HIV infection for non-injecting sexual partners'. *AIDS Care* **1,** 1. 51-58.

29. Philpot C.R., Harcourt C., Edwards J. and Grealis A. (1988) 'Human immunodeficiency virus and female prostitutes, Sydney 1985'. *Genitourin Med.* **64,** 193-197.

30. Farmer, R., Preston D., Emami J. and Barker M. (1989) *The Transmission of HIV with prisons and its likely effect on the growth of the epidemic in the general population.* Department of Community Medicine, Charing Cross and Westminster Medical School.

31. Harding T.W. (1987) 'Aids in Prison' *Lancet,* **ii.** 1260-1263

32. DOH (1989) *HIV and AIDS in prisons.* British Med. Assoc. Foundation for AIDS. Parliamentary Fact Sheet No. 7.

33. Curran L., McHugh M. and Nooney K. (1989) 'HIV Counselling in Prisons'. *AIDS Care.* **1,** 11-25.

34. MRC Medical Sociology Unit, University of Glasgow. *Work in Progress.* 1991.

35. Toomey K.E. and Cates W. (1989) 'Partner notification for the prevention of HIV infection'. *AIDS.* **3** 56-62.

36. Legal correspondent of the BMJ (1985) *Detaining patients with AIDS.* **291** 1102.

37. Brandt A.M. (1989) 'Four lessons from the History of Sexually Transmitted Diseases'. In: Promoting Safer Sex: International Workshop on the Prevention of Sexual Transmission of AIDS and other STD. *Amer. J. of Public Health.* 10-20. (30 April – 3 May)

38. Ohi G., Hasegawa T., Kai I., Inaba Y., Miyama T., Kamakura M., Terao H., Hirano W., Kobayashi Y., Muramatsu Y., Ashizawa M., Uemura I. and Niimi T. (1988) 'Notification of HIV Carriers: Possible effect on uptake of AIDS testing'. *Lancet,* Oct. 22. 947-949.

39. McEvoy M. (1987) 'Homosexual activity data in the United Kingdom'. In: *Future Trends in AIDS* p.89-96.

40. Duff C. and J.P. Hutchby (1988) 'Surveillance of AIDS cases: How acceptable are the figures'. *BMJ* **297** 965.

41. Peckham C.S., Tedder R.S., Briggs M., Ades A.E., Hjelm M., Wilcox A.H., Parra-Mejia N. and O'Connor C. (1990) 'Prevalence of maternal HIV infection based on unlinked anonymous testing of newborn babies'. *Lancet* **335**: 516-519.

42. The European Collaborative Study (1988) 'Mother-to-child transmission of HIV infection'. *Lancet* 5 Nov. 1039-1043

43. Lancet Editorial (1989) 'AIDS: Prevention, Policics, and Prostitutes'. *Lancet* **i,** 1111-1113.

44. Harcourt C., Philpot R. and Edwards J. (1989) 'The effects of condom use by clients on the incidence of STDs in female prostitutes' *Venereology* **2** 4-7.

45. Lancet Editorial (1990) 'Anonymous HIV testing' *Lancet* **335,** 575-576.

46. Coururier E., Brossard Y., Larsen C., Larsen M., Mazaubrun C. Du, Paris-Llado J., Gillot R., Henrion R., Breart G. and Brunet J.B. (1992 'HIV infection at outcome of pregnancy in the Paris area, France'. *Lancet* **340,** 707-709.

47. Knox E.G. (1991) 'Spatial and temporal studies in epidemiology' In: *Oxford Textbook of Public Health*. Second Edition. Volume 2, Methods of Public Health. Oxford 1991.

Acknowledgements

The main projects reported here, the survey of sexual behaviour and the development and application of a serviceable dynamic simulation model, were funded by the Medical Research Council. The initial studies of cervical cancer modelling from which this work was developed were conducted within a programme of health services research funded by the Department of Health. The authors would also like to thank Professor Ciaran Woodman, Ms Carole Cummins, Dr. Penny Blomfield, Ms. Mary Wardroper, Mrs. Clare Showell, Mr. Mark Bestell and Ms Hilary Kinnell for advice and assistance in developing the survey method and for additional information used in the report. We would like to thank Mr. Robert Lancashire for assistance with computer analyses and Anne Harvey, Sharon Murphy, Alison Green, Andrea Wright and Rachel Watkins for their help in the preparation of data files. We would like to thank Mrs. Sheila Allen and Mrs. Pam Wills for providing secretarial back-up throughout the whole project and Mrs. Sheila Allen for preparing the numerous drafts of this report.

Finally, we express our thanks, but cannot name, all of the organisations who gave access to their personnel and to our respondents themselves.

Printed in the United Kingdom for HMSO
Dd295542 2/93 C20 G531 10170